Psychoanalytic Work with Autistic Features in Adults

Psychoanalytic Work with Autistic Features in Adults deals with the diagnostic and therapeutic difficulties of working with patients with autistic residuals, formed in early life experiences that have remained dormant in the unconscious mind. Laura Tremelloni traces the process of identifying them in adult patients, and stresses the need to develop a treatment plan suitable for this kind of pathology.

This book uses clinical cases to examine the difficulties of work with hard to reach adults with 'gaps' in their sense of Self and symptoms related to primitive experiences of 'non-being'. Tremelloni presents new, adaptive therapeutic intervention methods for overcoming such obstacles and identifies the personification and permanence of undeveloped parts of the Self, in hard to reach adults who have otherwise developed satisfactorily and would not be diagnosed as autistic. In such cases, the author suggests the need for clinicians to adapt classic psychoanalytic approaches to the alternating levels of development of the separate parts which the Self has broken into.

Psychoanalytic Work with Autistic Features in Adults will help clinicians in psychoanalysis and psychoanalytic psychotherapy to more effectively reach such patients, whilst attempting to address the problematic limitations of therapeutic techniques in very difficult clinical cases.

Laura Tremelloni is a psychoanalytic psychotherapist in private practice in Milan, Italy, working particularly with autistic children and adults as well as psychotic patients. Her psychoanalytic training took place with analysts including Benedetti, Cremerius and McDougall, and then with Resnik, Tustin and Alvarez. She is a founding member of the Centro Internazionale Studi Psicodinamici della Personalità (CISPP), Venice, with Salomon Resnik and other colleagues, where lessons, seminars and meetings are held regularly, especially on infantile autism and psychosis.

Psychoanalytic Work with Autistic Features in Adults

Clinical Intervention Methods and Technique

Laura Tremelloni

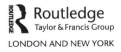

LONDON AND NEW YORK

First published 2018
by Routledge
2 Park Square, Milton Park, Abingdon, Oxon OX14 4RN

and by Routledge
711 Third Avenue, New York, NY 10017

Routledge is an imprint of the Taylor & Francis Group, an informa business

© 2018 Laura Tremelloni

The right of Laura Tremelloni to be identified as author of this work has been asserted by her in accordance with sections 77 and 78 of the Copyright, Designs and Patents Act 1988.

All rights reserved. No part of this book may be reprinted or reproduced or utilised in any form or by any electronic, mechanical, or other means, now known or hereafter invented, including photocopying and recording, or in any information storage or retrieval system, without permission in writing from the publishers.

Translated into English by Giuliana Di Gregorio and Camilla Gamba

Trademark notice: Product or corporate names may be trademarks or registered trademarks, and are used only for identification and explanation without intent to infringe.

British Library Cataloguing-in-Publication Data
A catalogue record for this book is available from the British Library

Library of Congress Cataloging-in-Publication Data
Names: Tremelloni, Laura, author.
Title: Psychoanalytic work with autistic features in adults: clinical intervention methods and technique / Laura Tremelloni.
Description: Abingdon, Oxon; New York, NY: Routledge, 2018. | Includes bibliographical references and index.
Identifiers: LCCN 2017060117 (print) | LCCN 2017060652 (ebook) | ISBN 9781351014595 (Master) | ISBN 9781351014588 (Web PDF) | ISBN 9781351014571 (ePub) | ISBN 9781351014564 (Mobipocket/Kindle) | ISBN 9781138497788 (hbk: alk. paper) | ISBN 9781138497801 (pbk : alk. paper) | ISBN 9781351014595 (ebk)
Subjects: | MESH: Autistic Disorder–therapy | Adult | Autistic Disorder–psychology | Psychoanalytic Therapy–methods
Classification: LCC RC553.A88 (ebook) | LCC RC553.A88 (print) | NLM WM 203.5 | DDC 616.85/882–dc23
LC record available at https://lccn.loc.gov/2017060117

ISBN: 978-1-138-49778-8 (hbk)
ISBN: 978-1-138-49780-1 (pbk)
ISBN: 978-1-351-01459-5 (ebk)

Typeset in Times New Roman
by Wearset Ltd, Boldon, Tyne and Wear

In memory of Salomon Resnik,
Whose human warmth and richness of thought inspired to continue my search for new meanings.
To him, a fond memory and my complete gratitude for the generosity with which he shared his experience as a brave and original psychoanalyst.

I dedicate this book to my sons, Francesco and Fabio, and to my grandchildren, Tommaso, Fiammetta, Samuele and Olivia, with love.

Contents

Preface: explorations in terra incognita — ix
Acknowledgements — xiii

Introduction — 1

PART I — 5
1 About autism — 7
2 About skin: the skin as a surface of the body — 26
3 About sight and beauty — 38

PART II — 49
4 Clinical examples — 51
5 Sara: living on the surface — 55
6 Irene: from robot-like to person — 94
7 Beatriz: backwards love — 102
8 Monica: the psychic retreat — 109

PART III — 115
9 First encounters: adventures into the unknown — 117
10 Transference and countertransference — 121
11 The challenges of working with autistic traits — 132

12 Suggestions for therapeutic interventions	138
Conclusions	154
Index	156

Preface
Explorations in terra incognita

The aim of this book is to bring together analytic work that has been carried out over many years in order to show the importance of our thoughts and observations regarding our patients' problems, as well as our own, with the intention of mitigating their existential difficulties and symptoms.

The result of analytic work can be astonishing and even comforting, as we are able to lead our patients to imagine new possibilities for fulfilment. On the other hand, if the relationship is interrupted before our work comes to an end – indicating that the relationship has broken down – we have to reflect upon what, how and why we failed to understand.

We may wonder why psychoanalysts write so much about their clinical cases. The simplest answer is that these written cases reflect their desire to share their experience of analytic psychotherapy with their colleagues, or to add to a theoretical discussion.

As a matter of fact, when put to paper, analytic work becomes imperfect and artificial: the totality of thoughts, associations, feelings and details is left out. Although all these things cannot be retrieved and described, they exist as a whole in our mind. This totality follows the changes within the patient, within our relationship and even within ourselves.

How can one convey that a single word pronounced by the patient might evoke in the therapist an emotion or a memory, which in turn connects with the intention of the patient and thus leads to an interpretation?

In testifying to the value of psychoanalytic work, the written word as a 'set of signs' is not a mere vehicle of information regarding the analytic journey. The word must also transmit the emotions felt by both participants as well as the way they interconnect. What happens in the analyst's consulting room involves a particular encounter between two people that leads to a new, unexpected relationship. This marks the beginning of a third new situation.

When we speak of the vicissitudes of the transference and highlight our encounter with the primitive and unconscious parts of ourselves, something inevitably emerges through spoken word and body language. Therefore, in writing about psychoanalytic work, the analyst can neither avoid self-reference nor keep from displaying unconscious signs of personal enigmas.

In fact, no description of the vicissitudes of the analytic journey, however accurate, precise and sincere it may be, can accurately portray what really transpires between the analyst and the patient: the emotions, the sensations, the atmosphere of the sessions and its variability. Our memory can relate facts but it cannot bring us to relive the intensity of our feelings. How can we then transmit through our writing our emotions and the links and personal associations that intensify these emotions? How can the written word convey the state of attentive listening regarding the particular subject being discussed? How can we demonstrate the trajectory of the work that leads to a positive outcome? Why do so many psychoanalysts write about their work? Is it simply a matter of narcissistic exhibitionism?

Françoise Gantheret (2010), a French psychoanalyst and novelist, asserts that writing about psychoanalytic work denotes 'the nostalgia of the present': the emotions of that fleeting moment of life suddenly disappear and leave a void. Emotions represent our present: writing about them at a later moment is a way of bringing them back to life, wishing time hadn't moved forward.

I, however, believe that in describing clinical cases, we take back possession of time that has passed and we can once again experience important fragments of the life we shared with the patient. In fact, writing is our attempt to overcome our feelings of loss and nostalgia related to the past experience of having had a profound encounter with another person.

Writing about psychoanalytic cases also pushes us to think back over our life through our patients' vicissitudes.

When we meet a patient for the first time, we find ourselves faced with an unknown world, of which we perceive only the external image. We obtain real and immediate information from the body, its movements and posture, as well as the voice and the content of what is being said. We begin to imagine an internal world that we understand through our own way of feeling and thinking. Moreover, we find ourselves faced with incomprehensible, mysterious elements. Gradually and over time, new elements come into our internal imagined landscape so that the initial picture becomes increasingly more complex and raises new questions. Our personal way of being intersects with the patient's personality.

The gradual understanding of the patient's personality can be compared to the discovery of a new continent. This leads me back to the time I visited the French National Library in Paris for an exhibition on the cartography of the African continent. Just like the continuous transformation of graphic maps over time, our own understanding of the patient changes gradually over time during the course of analysis. We experience discoveries and marvels, wrong turns and disappointments, agreement and misunderstanding, personal discoveries and new thoughts.

I was fascinated by the reproduction of original maps. By sailing repeatedly across the surrounding seas, the ancient Greeks observed the shapes of the areas explored. They began to create mental representations of the contours of the inlets in order to place them on the map.

The distances and the shapes were correlated with the means of transport of the time – that is, rowing boats. During the era of Tolomeo (second century AD), the shape of Africa was thus only represented in its northern part, near the Mediterranean, while the southern part did not exist and was termed '*terra incognita*'.

After this period, we have no records of further interest in new geographical discoveries. It wasn't until the sixteenth century that interest in the world and the shape of maps was renewed: maps portraying the celestial sphere were parallel to those representing the world.

When men went beyond the limits of the Mediterranean, they began exploring new areas, identifying new lands and giving them new names, occupying and colonizing new territories by going into battle. This led to rivalries among conquerors. The exploration of new areas quickly turned into a craving for possession and led to additional conflicts.

Interest in the first maps was expressed through a mix of information gathered through sailing experiences and the invention of places and imaginary elements. For example, different animals such as lions and giraffes, at the time still unknown, were drawn in the middle of the continent. Other fantastic animals and landmarks, such as flying fish or imaginary mountains and islands, were invented and added. The mix of information that emerged from experience and imagination gradually gave birth to the first real map. We can thus see the graphic representation of what is real and what is imagined.

The act of drawing maps evidently came after each discovery. The new name given to a territory symbolized the birth of a new land, and the act of conquest was thus placed on the map. The original name of the map of the world was: '*teatrum orbis terrarum, teatrum mundis*'.

Before current technological discoveries, cartography was considered to be 'an art form between reductive abstraction and an aesthetic appropriation' (Schalansky, 2010). For example, as it was impossible to represent the rounded shape of the Earth on paper, it became flat; these projections altered the representation of the world, and the representations altered the measurements. Cartography changed from the study and knowledge of visible elements to the need to give them shape and reduce the measurements of the land.

In a rather troubling story by Jorge Luis Borges (1999), during the Ming Dynasty (1368–1644) some cartographers who were intent on representing a very detailed map of the limitless Chinese empire ended up creating a map describing the empire on a 1:1 scale. This was a paradoxical attempt to combine two overlapping dimensions: the representation of an object and the object being represented. The result was an enormous map representing the extent of the empire, transformed into condensed spaces.

Much in the same way, we approach and try to get to know a new patient by adding our own fantasies and perceptions to their version of themselves. Gradually, we both come to acknowledge that there is an inner space, and we start to discover what had before been unseen.

I think that geographical discoveries can be compared with analytic work: we can discover places like the Garden of Eden and its hidden treasures, or barren lands, or bellicose populations.

Does 'terra incognita' represent the unconscious mind described in psychoanalytic theory?

In our mind, the image of the patient is formed through perceptions, intuitions, evidence, associations and feelings elicited by the mix of transference and countertransference. This image is a subjective and arbitrary construction, which changes during the analysis, partly as a consequence of new thoughts and interpretations. The discovery of previously unknown areas and connections between areas that have already been explored can lead the patient to experience internal conflicts, as well as external conflicts with the explorer-analyst. The patient comes to understand and acknowledge unknown parts of his or her personality, and reduces other structures that had previously characterized a problematic past.

I would like to draw here an analogy between geographical discoveries and narcissistic certainties: though these initially represent safe havens, through analytic work they can become places of disappointment and depression.

The personality also holds islands in which primitive autistic experiences prevent the development of affective life.

These are the territories that I propose to explore here with the readers.

References

Borges, J. L. (1999) *Collected fictions*, translated by Andrew Hurley, London: Penguin Random House.

Gantheret, F. (2010) *La nostalgie du present*, Paris: Editions de l'Olivier.

Schalansky, J. (2010) *Atllas des iles abandonnées*, Paris: Artaud, Flammarion.

Acknowledgements

I would like to thank my patients, who have been able to trust in me when faced with long and arduous paths, even before developing new hope for their lives. They helped me in my reflections regarding myself.

This book would not have come to light without the observations and support of Judith Edwards and the priceless considerations of Anne Alvarez, who I thank with great gratitude and esteem.

I must also thank my colleagues of the CISPP Venice Group for listening to my questions and offering fertile feedback.

In particular, thank you to Isabella Schiappadori, who shared the moments of doubts and difficulties that arose during my therapeutic work. Her generous observations have always led to new points of view.

I want to thank my sons, Francesco and Fabio, who have always helped me in my efforts to write about my experiences; my grandchildren, Tommaso and Fiammetta, who have pulled me out of technical difficulties; and Simona and Valeria for their affectionate participation.

I would also like to thank Giuliana Di Gregorio and Camilla Gamba, who have overseen the English edition of this work with passion and competence.

Introduction

The fascination of the analyst's work consists in the plurality of the questions that arise from our patients' personalities. Initially, the structures of the Self and the various pathological forms drive us to measure ourselves with what we know and face our current personal dilemmas.

The terms related to the realm of autism, such as the expression 'autistic features', used in the title, may raise questions or create diagnostic confusion. I'd like to clarify that the adult patients discussed here do not appear to be pathological on the surface, but have hidden parts of the Self that have been uninhabited; I have defined these hidden parts in my previous work as 'capsules/nuclei/autistic residues' containing primitive experiences that have been left unknown (Tremelloni, 2005). These subjects have gaps in the Self and show symptoms linked to primitive experiences of non-being. These non-mentalized nuclei are inaccessible to feelings and have been buried in the unconscious; they can remain dormant within the personality until they manifest through the explosion of psychotic or psychosomatic symptoms, which may emerge during significant personal events (Klein, 1980; Tustin, 1986; Tremelloni, 2005, Barrows, 2008).

In some cases, acute psychotic breakdowns expose the existence of these primitive and painful affective experiences, which had never before been acknowledged by the patient. These can be noted in the absence of affective exchanges with the analyst and picked up through the countertransference.

The aim of this book is primarily to illustrate the type of analytic work needed to identify these parts and to shed light on the changes that can be made to therapeutic interventions. Here I describe the search for new approaches, 'created and invented on the spot', based on the patient's peculiarities and the countertransference, in order to overcome obstacles and reach out to the patient who has become entrenched within his or her armour.

In particular, I describe in detail two cases in which the suffering was manifested through the skin; I look into the relationship between the skin and early sensory experiences that impact the construction of the Self. The other cases refer to borderline patients for whom primitive experiences of emotional suffering were hidden behind a mask of 'normality'.

My main purpose is to highlight the process of analytic work in relation to the presence and discovery of these parts. In order to overcome the obstacles and reach patients who are enclosed in their armour, we have to find new ways of moving forward.

I will try to describe the necessary alterations to therapeutic interventions, 'created in the moment' in accordance with our feelings. These alterations pose the problematic issue of the meaning and limits of 'technique' in psychoanalytic psychotherapy, which in this case is linked to both clinical experience and the analyst's personality.

My working hypothesis is based on the fact that I have encountered patients with these characteristics who had previously undergone long psychoanalyses, yet had not seen any changes; this was due to the fact that these primitive nuclei had not been identified and therefore analysed. These autistic nuclei remain dormant in the personality until they are awakened by the explosion of psychological or psychosomatic symptoms. Significant life events can trigger such crises. The presence of these capsules can reveal itself at the beginning of the work through the lack of emotional involvement the individual displays towards the analyst.

There is a need to adapt ways of intervening at different moments in the relationship, by following the vicissitudes of the transference and the countertransference. These variations are also determined by the stage of integration of the Self and the different degrees to which the patient can symbolize.

Psychoanalytic work with children or adults who have autistic nuclei that lie far from affective relationships is challenging. The obstacles I have encountered in my work have driven me to reconsider what my colleagues have thought and theorized in similar situations. Each author provides us with different points of view to investigate and evaluate, and this in turn leads to new questions and thoughts. When I think about my favourite teachers (the ones I have had the privilege to know personally or those who I have known only through their writings), I hold imaginary conversations with them: I then feel reassured about the journey I'm on and find it easier to tolerate the frustration of not knowing how to proceed. The memory of my interactions with these people whom I consider to have been my mentors always helps me think and hope.

In the same way, at times, I am comforted by the thought of my patients who come to see the profound changes they have made despite having faced extreme hardships in their lives. After many years of analysis, they move from primitive and frozen emotional states to experiencing the possibility of feeling alive as human beings.

These occasions of comfort have filled me with the enthusiasm to carry on my therapeutic work (even in extremely complex situations), as well as continue my own psychoanalysis. As we try to clarify the meaning and the development of a pathological state such as autism or psychosis, we discover that we ourselves have had similar – albeit transient and less significant – childhood experiences.

We must always remember that being a psychoanalyst means being both patient and therapist, without neglecting the responsibility of our role. From the very beginning of my work, I have always been aware of the danger of wearing the mask of the omniscient and completely neutral analyst, detached from the complexity of reality and my own emotions. How one is and feels as a psychoanalyst will change during the course of a lifetime, and will involve our own personal transformations as well as changes in our ideas.

First we have to uncover the patient's true quest that lies beneath the formal referral or diagnosis. An element that I have found in some of the patients I describe here is a lack of passion or emotional closeness that is present from the moment an individual asks for psychoanalysis; this is an indication of the difficult human relationship that is about to commence. Over time, a lack of mental integration preventing a real sense of existence becomes evident.

I remember that J. McDougall (1989) described her difficulties in working psychoanalytically with patients she called 'desaffectés', those who had cut off feelings from their inner world as a result of primitive emotional experiences.

Bion (1970) considers that some patients feel pain, but without suffering. Emotional suffering is not experienced internally as a mental state; it is anaesthetized and can be expressed through adequate words – as though it were a script – but it is not accompanied by an emotional experience. On the other hand, if projected externally, this emotional suffering is experienced as hostility instigated by the other. Thus, the difficulty in reaching the patient emerges. It is difficult to establish an interpersonal relationship that can represent a real experience of communication and mental unity.

The lengthy duration of these therapies could be seen as a sign of failure or passivity of the treatment: failure on the part of both the patient and the psychoanalyst. On the contrary, when there is an autistic primitive experience, the length of the analytic relationship is a true privilege for both parties. Time allows both patient and psychoanalyst to maintain hope for consistent and previously inconceivable developments of mental and affective states.

I will describe in detail patients with deficits in the Self. The part of the Self which is essentially one of 'not-being' is difficult to identify and connect with. To do so requires lengthy therapeutic work, which differs in its various stages. Other cases, however, reveal the intensity of unexpected yet authentic and exciting encounters.

Content

The main theme of this work concerns the process of personification and the permanence of undeveloped parts of the Self in adults who have had a more or less satisfactory overall development.

Starting with Sara's case, which is described in detail, I will discuss the concept of body image and the importance of the skin in the experiences of autistic states. I will also look at failure in the process of symbolization, which normally derives from physical and emotional experiences in early childhood.

In order to accurately illustrate the complexity of each individual, while at the same time protecting their anonymity, the clinical cases presented here are a collage of partially similar situations.

The psychoanalytic trajectory of these cases illustrates the need to adapt interventions at various points during the therapy in order to follow the vicissitudes of the transference relationship. These changes are also linked to the analyst's as well as to the patient's own variable ability to symbolize.

About confidentiality

Confidentiality remains an ongoing concern in any therapeutic relationship. In all medical fields, the description and discussion of clinical cases is used to increase knowledge and to propose new therapeutic prospects to be published for the purpose of teaching others. These descriptions should not come to represent exercises in narcissism either by the patient or by the therapist. The clinical cases described here are intended to illustrate long and complex therapeutic journeys that I would like to submit to clinical discussion.

In order to preserve the anonymity of the individuals involved, I have modified names and circumstances. I have also eliminated or changed some biographical details at the risk of making some links and connections unclear to the reader. As explained above, these 'collages' are meant to preserve the anonymity of the work. In my opinion, it is preferable for the reader to feel perplexed at times than for the author to reveal details of confidential work.

References

Barrows, K. (2008) *Autism in childhood and autistic features in adults*, London: Karnac.
Bion, W. (1970) *Attention and interpretation*, London: Tavistock Publications.
Klein, S. (1980) 'Autistic phenomena in neurotic patients', *International Journal of Psychoanalysis*, 61, 395–401.
McDougall, J. (1989) 'One body for two'. In *Theaters of the body* (pp. 140–161), London: Free Association Books.
Tremelloni, L. (2005) *Arctic spring: potential for growth in adults with psychosis and autism*, London: Karnac.
Tustin, F. (1986) *Autistic barriers in neurotic patients*, London: Karnac.

Part I

Chapter 1

About autism

1.1 Autistic traits and features in adults

Starting from the 1970s, following studies on autism in children, several authors began discussing adult patients with traces of autism (Winnicott, 1960; Rosenfeld, 1979, 1987; Klein, 1980; Tustin, 1986; Ogden, 1989; Mitrani, 1996; Tremelloni, 2005; Barrows, 2008; Civitarese, 2013). These patients are characterized by having a part of the Self that is sufficiently developed to conduct an apparently 'normal' social life, while another part of the Self has remained incomplete due to a defective development of the process of symbolization.

In psychoanalytic work, the analyst is faced with patients who are initially considered to be neurotic or borderline. She then realizes that it is impossible to establish any form of real communication with them. This difficulty is due, in part, to a lack of personal meanings in their thoughts, due to a lack of symbolization, and in part to the avoidance of emotional contact, which is a trace of early psychological suffering. The primitive emotional suffering dates back to the foetal period and to the very first years of life. This pain was perceived on a sensory and affective level and recorded in the unconscious mind; it remains unknown. It is part of the non-represented material and is kept in the implicit memory. Mancia (2003) holds that this material kept in the unconscious mind can be traced in the process of psychoanalysis only through the patient's dreams and transference.

During their early development, these subjects have buried more or less intense or extensive experiences of autistic states, alternated with schizo-paranoid mental states. This alternating of mental states comes to light during the course of psychoanalytical work. This primitive pain may also reveal itself in cases of psychosis.

The only possible communication in the analytical relationship can take place in the intuition of the pain and the emotional needs of the patients, which the analyst can perceive through her countertransference and reverie.

In a previous publication (Tremelloni, 2005), I traced the history of the term 'autism' used in psychiatry, and I described the autistic residuals as 'capsules' or 'autistic nuclei'. This concept refers to a more or less extended psychic area which contains traces of primitive autistic reactions to extreme childhood anxiety and sensory experiences that have not been processed. These encapsulated parts of the personality can remain hidden under psychosomatic personalities or neurotic, psychotic or borderline psychological organizations.

Identifying this type of pathology is key to ensuring that the psychoanalytical intervention is appropriate for the individual's degree of development of the Self.

1.2 Searching for non-mentalized experiences

The reflections of this work relate to therapy with adult patients who have developed a partially neurotic, psychotic or borderline psychological structure, which may or may not have already been analysed. As a result of emotionally significant events, these patients experience sudden episodes of terror and show signs of personality disintegration.

As I have already indicated, this occurrence was described and studied by many authors in the second half of the last century. Linking the origins of such symptoms in early life experiences, Bion (1962) speaks of children who have known 'nameless dread'. Winnicott (1971a) believes the fear of mental breakdown derives from primitive anxieties that re-emerge as a result of the environment's inability to meet the child's needs. Tustin (1986) speaks of 'uncontrollable unnamed terror', 'states of non-experience' and 'the black hole'. Grotstein (1990a) describes the experience of the 'black hole' as a frightening sense of lack of power and 'non-existence', or as a centripetal force towards emptiness. He specifies the subject feels that there is no human presence in the space outside the Self, or rather, that there is a malevolent and inhuman absence.

These archaic and sensory-dominated experiences are defined as 'unmentalized' (Mitrani, 2008) because they have occurred prior to the child's ability to symbolize. In my previous work, I defined these early experiences as 'autistic-type capsules', and described how they remain buried in the Self until they are identified and acknowledged later on in life (Tremelloni, 2005).

Given the degree of Ego development that has enabled these patients to reach a satisfactory level of social relations, it is difficult to imagine that these individuals possess a frail and needy Self. This situation confuses the analyst who, caught between the false Self and the true Self, cannot discern a real request for help. Due to their early emotional fragility, the efforts of such people have been directed towards the construction of a solid personality and a robust set of skills.

However, in the early stages of contact, one may notice certain peculiarities in the relational distance, such as the individual's inability to acknowledge the difference in roles, an excessive familiarity, a lack of discretion or tactlessness. This highlights the fact that there is very little awareness of boundaries and personal space. Moreover, such people manifest a deficit in the process of symbolization and attribution of meaning.

Premature encapsulation contains primitive emotional experiences that have been frozen and buried in the unconscious within rigid structures; they are hidden behind defences that have been erected for psychic survival. Because these individuals do not undergo the process of self-development, they remain static and enclosed in a strong armour that protects from 'feeling'. In these early experiences, there is a persistent lack of trust regarding stable emotional relationships, but there is also a positive and vital potential.

By paying attention to changes in the transference and countertransference, we can pick up the existence of autistic experiences from subliminal signs, which we perceive in the fluctuating emotional contact. Thus, in an attempt to track these primitive experiences, we can follow different paths, trying to emerge from the confusion brought on by the patient's intertwined defensive responses.

The pervasive anxiety of these first encounters can be masked by great self-confidence, different degrees of mania and lack of doubt regarding the meanings of the stories these individuals bring to the analyst. One may be surprised by a tendency to deny that there is any anxiety in meeting the analyst: the patient may appear to be festive and jovial as one would be with old friends. Other times, the overbearing part of the personality emerges in an attempt to fill the void left by emotional deprivation.

One may come across delusional ideation or troubling physical symptoms: the focus tends to be on the body as the place of primitive conflicts and confusion between the Self and the other. The concepts of closeness, distance, separation and individuation have not been processed and thus create anxiety.

As communication progresses, the pathological situation becomes more evident; the patient enters a state of acute crisis and experiences a sense of disorientation and confusion about the Self, leading to a more or less explicit request for a fusional relationship with the analyst.

The experience of non-differentiation accompanied by high levels of anxiety confirms the re-emergence of primitive experiences, which may include the lack of corporal boundaries, the terror of falling into a limitless and formless space, and the absence of a relationship with an object able to support and contain the individual.

In such cases, the beginning and the course of the psychoanalytic process are riddled with difficulties in the transference; this signals the re-enactment in the relationship with the analyst of the crippling experiences of loneliness, lack of trust and persecutory fears.

When the moment of crisis seems to be overcome, the analytic relationship becomes once again very difficult, albeit in different ways. This is due to the pathological personality structure. The destructive feelings attached to these autistic experiences cause various defences to be erected and consolidated, confusing the analyst.

These defences vary and can be represented by intellectual constructs in which words are detached from feelings; they are autistic objects not aimed at communication, but rather at exhibition. In the case of a patient of mine, an aspiring writer, my words were scrambled and repeated in literary productions and intellectual formulations: these productions were more akin to imitation than to the internalization that characterizes an evolutionary process. The compositions masked a rejection of real emotional contact with the theft of a few valuable elements from my words.

At other times, what prevails may be excessive projective identification, used to eliminate persecutory anxieties or feelings of anger. Such defences prevent the analyst from seeing the patient's need for help, and this hinders the analytic work. The need for help is projected onto the other, prompting the mask of altruism, a denial of one's own aggressive feelings through seductive or falsely generous behaviour.

Another solution the patient uses with regards to the pain of reconsidering the entirety of his or her life story is escaping into mania or humour, transforming painful feelings into excitement or sadistic attacks. Another solution may be an actual escape from analysis through a sudden interruption.

Narcissism is another important obstacle to the development of thought in analysis; it may be so strong that it does not allow one to listen to the other. Other forms of defence may be: the persistence of psychosomatic symptoms and hypochondriac states; an obsessive mode of thought which prevents any transformation; the use of acting-out, especially in the forms of substance abuse or sexual behaviour.

In conclusion, when faced with the difficulties that arise from the inability to work with free associations or attribution of meanings, linking thoughts with discontinuous affective behaviour, countertransference remains the principal therapeutic research tool.

1.3 Non-represented mental states[1]

My interest in primitive non-mentalized states initially arose from my clinical work with children with autism, and later with adult patients who, while seeming potentially analysable, manifested specific difficulties in taking up classical analytical work through personal affective communication.

To listen analytically means to continually integrate contents with their temporal and logical connections, and with the feelings aroused in the analyst. All this is also linked to his or her theoretical background. The development of the traditional analytic discourse is hindered by the difficulty in establishing these links, along with a reduced affective relationship and a communicative vacuum. On one hand, the analyst is faced with the patient's suffering; on the other he or she must deal with the impossibility of establishing a connection between the current anxiety and the story that is being remembered and recounted.

These clinical experiences moved me to search for theoretical explanations. Starting from the work of Alvarez, Bion, Green, Sidney Klein, Ogden, Tustin and Winnicott, several recent studies have broadened my theoretical understanding of these issues in order to come up with some therapeutic changes.[2]

The representational ability is the result of the psyche's active primordial work in dealing with internal stimuli (drives) and external stimuli (perceptions).

The psyche will gradually organize itself through the establishment of the object relationship, the memory of different emotional experiences, the repetitions or changes of the surrounding environmental events and their interconnections. The ability to represent the absent object will allow the development of thinking (Freud, 1913; O'Shaughnessy, 1964). The non-neurotic patients we are discussing, however, are unable to represent a primary object (Reed, 2009).

The representation of the absent object shows how the ability to think enables the mind to hold onto what is not directly perceived in a given moment in the surrounding space.

Non-represented mental states are a sign of a representational deficit linked to traumatic experiences in a pre-verbal period that have led to autistic or psychotic nuclei. These are evident in states of anguish and emptiness: they are impossible to describe, they can be expressed through action and not through words, they reduce the ability to link thoughts with feelings.

Reed (2006, 2009) reflections are an elaboration of the contributions of Green and Winnicott. Green (1983a, 1986, 1993, 1997, 1998, 2002) initially addressed the issue of non-represented states in his work with adult patients. In his work on the dead mother (1983b), he suggests that in these cases the identification with the mother is a representation of the absence of representation. One can think of it as an empty mirror in which the patient loses his reflection. This unconscious identification that cannot be translated into language remains unrepresented in the unconscious.

For Green, the representation of the primary object takes place only if a vital instinct prevails over the death drive and the withdrawal of object investments. In non-representation, the conflict is to be found between investment and the creative power of love that unites a baby to life on one hand, and the death drive on the other, which leads to a withdrawal of that investment. The latter case has a de-objectifying function (Spitz, 1965; Green, 2002), meaning a disconnection from any search for meaning. When the internal tension provokes a strong dissatisfaction, the defence aroused to quell the tension causes the renunciation of the object, and all is obliterated: this is the vacuum that Green calls negative hallucination. In this vacuum there is no perception of an object or of a perceptible psychic phenomenon; it is the equivalent of a loss of meaning.

Green highlighted the vacuum in these patients' symbolic representations. If the vacuum holds something that can neither be expressed through words nor even be thought, the transference happens through the object rather than through the use of words. Words are thus used to express instinctual needs and are therefore devoid of specific meaning: they express the need for a transitional object to act as a real object.

From a therapeutic point of view, if the vacuum represents the residue of the solution to past conflicts, the patient looks to the current setting for what was missing in the past: that is, someone to pay attention to him, to listen to him, to take pleasure in being with him, to offer verbal explanations so that he may invest positively in a less disappointing transitional object.

When the patient has to face an unpleasant external reality, he reacts with variable internal states and a repetition of a partial and irregular dis-investment, expressed in the current moment.

The lack of a backdrop on which to fantasize is a defence mechanism that obliterates what could be an unconscious internal world. Other defences that may later emerge to evade an absence of meaning may include seemingly nonsensical outbursts; actions that are not supported by any form of ideation; a retreat into depression; self-harming behaviour connected to repeated frustrations; and various addictions and somatic symptoms.

One feature common to these subjects is the lack of continuity on an affective level. The Self is felt to be worthless and is fused with the devalued object; thus it is un-usable or hostile. These patients fear abandonment and need affection, but if one comes too close to them, they feel invaded and retract out of fear of encountering a persecutory object. Another part of the Self is imagined to be omnipotent, or even critical and judgemental. Thus, one experiences a paralysis of affect and feeling along with the return of the same suffering and the same behaviour.

The failure to identify with the object can also lead to decreased ability to create representations, symbolize, and make free associations and connections between thoughts (Bion, 1970).

In clinical practice we find patients who, though they may experience professional success, remain bound to primitive anxieties and fears regarding abandonment and relationships that are too close. They refuse relationships, they may isolate themselves and are prone to depression; there is an almost hallucinatory presence in the Self of bad objects, and they tend to idealize.

Winnicott (1953, 1971a, 1971b, 1971c, 1974) stressed the importance of the object, the transitional space and the object's primary function in supporting and enhancing the process of taking in reality. The object's role is to mediate the development of meanings: its prolonged absence determines the failure of meanings. If the mother is too often absent, the internal representation fades and the transitional phenomena become meaningless. For the construction of the Self and the object representation to take place, the object must behave in such a way so as to not only meet the child's needs, but also be present through time and be constant in the child's mental state.

The object representation is achieved through the union of instinct and meaning. Traces of bodily tension followed by the feeling of satisfaction connected to an affective object are bound together in memory. If, however, the representation of the object is not linked to satisfaction and pleasure because the object is absent, distant or erratic, one experiences the fading away of the representation and of its memory (Reed, 2009).

In order to work with patients who bring these states of suffering, the analyst has to regress to childhood emotional states of suffering in order to find a means of communication that both can understand, and share the angst experienced by both (Tremelloni, 2005).

With regard to the concept of representation, Botella and Botella (2005) introduced the term *figurability* to indicate a new ability to give shape and meaning to experiences of a primitive period of the individual's life, when these experiences could not yet be represented. This can be considered to be a creative ability: it sheds light on the fact that the suffering comes from non-represented states which had hitherto been hidden.

1.4 The black hole[3]

In my analytic work, I have found that these adults who have had primitive traumatic experiences are haunted by a feeling of falling into a black hole. They are filled with angst that has no apparent explanation in their minds, nor in that of the analyst.

The expression 'black hole' was introduced in psychoanalysis by Tustin (1972, 1986, 1990, 1992) and by Grotstein (1986, 1989, 1990a, 1990b, 1990c, 1993), after Bion (1970) – who had been their analyst – described the experience of childhood catastrophe in psychotics, caused by early experiences of lack of support and meaning. Bion talks about a 'nameless dread' in the child that arises when the child projects onto the mother a fear of death, and the mother is unable to hold this projection and transmit it back to the baby in a bearable form.

In her work with autistic children, Tustin (1972) interpreted the expression of falling into a 'black hole' used by a young patient as a metaphor for a subjective experience of falling into a dark and terrifying space. According to the author, this experience derives from an early disconnection with a mother who had been initially believed to be part of the child's own body. The black hole thus represents experiences of unbearable rupture, black depression, despair, rage, terror, helplessness and hopelessness.

Similarly, Winnicott (1960) talked of *annihilation anxiety* in his work 'The theory of the parent-infant relationship'. With reference to adult psychotic and borderline patients, Grotstein (1990a) applies this term to indicate primitive experiences characterized by an endless, bottomless, meaningless space, an experience of nothingness, disorganization, chaos and nameless dread. The phenomenon of the black hole thus represents one of the frightening aspects of initial fears of annihilation in human life. Grotstein holds that the black hole represents the death instinct and signals the failure of a healthy attachment in early development. The experience is that of a terrifying weakness, helplessness, nothingness, non-existence.

Grotstein links this mental state to the concept of 'black holes' in astrophysics. He describes the experience of the 'black hole' not as a static vacuum but as a space in which an implosive centripetal force is at work. The hole stands for the depths of the emptiness that contains unacknowledged parts of the psyche. The black quality symbolizes the death of meanings of the Self and of objects. This space is not an area in which human relationships can develop; it holds an un-human and malevolent absence that must be kept from consciousness. Thus, an altered and perverse reconstruction of the subjective world invades the world of the psychotic person.

Edwards (1994) used this same astrophysics concept in her work with an adolescent patient. She described the black hole in her patient's mind as a fear of annihilation and of falling into a limitless space.

There are many strategies to avoid these experiences of destruction, their objective being to eliminate impending past catastrophic experiences: hence, various defences are erected. The black hole is a psychological disaster; in other words, it is a defective formation of the Self. The experience of nothingness and lack of meaning differs from mentalized experiences as such, if considered in relation to a future moment. In addition to the damaging primitive experiences of nothingness, we have here an accumulation of 'non-things' and 'non-matter'. The bizarre behaviour of psychotics is due to particular defences and attempts to keep from falling into the black hole.

Grotstein (1987) emphasizes that, for borderline patients, the difficulty in experiencing change in analysis arises from the fact that immobile immature aspects in the Self persistently obstruct the constructive and innovative activity of the other part of the Self that strives for new developments.

Subsequently, Eshel (1998) extended the metaphorical meaning of the black hole to the phenomena described in psychoanalysis. Unlike Tustin and Grotstein, this author interprets the phenomenon of the black hole as an interpersonal and intra-psychic space dominated by a central object that has been experienced as a black hole. A shadow permeates this psychic space and hinders any emotional closeness in subjects who have otherwise developed normal social and professional lives. Eshel believes that the black hole of the psychic world has an internal gravitational force powerful enough to encompass everything that approaches it, as in the astrophysics notion.

Based on my experience with patients who have 'fallen into the black hole' at different moments of the analysis, I agree with Eshel's view that every new experience of emotional closeness recalls primitive experiences and impedes any change in the Self. Thus, one can experience emotional contact with the patient one moment, only to see him or her pull violently away the next.

For this reason, these analyses take a long time and aim to bring the patient away from the attraction of that inner destructiveness and paralysis that pervades all affective communication. This new experience of permanence in a space that had previously been devoid of time and space coordinates may help explain the difficulty these individuals have in respecting time and modulating distance and space in interpersonal contact.

In the stories told by some of my patients, the experiences of the black hole can be connected to various forms of neglect on behalf of the mother – for example, due to her emotional or physical absence in cases of bereavement, having to look after family members with disabilities, more or less severe mental or physical illnesses, extreme poverty, or – finally – violence.

1.5 Attachment and affective distance

Attachment theory, first proposed and elaborated on by Bowlby (1986), highlights the need to establish a solid bond between two living beings. This may take the form of an object-related bond of dependency or a symbiotic stage prior to individuation. The child needs physical closeness and contact with a being who can ensure his or her survival and maintain internal homeostasis. This human being must be part of a loving relationship, which manifests itself through closeness and presence, allowing also for subsequent separation. Attachment is a pattern of behaviour that provides a feeling of security and regulates the emotional experience. Separation anxiety is the inevitable and natural response of the child when the mother moves away.

Attachment is not only superficial contact of the skin; it is a point of reference between the skin of two people that gives rise to the experience of distance or closeness. The awareness of proximity is initially a physical awareness, and then becomes emotional. The concept of proximity later takes on the broader meaning of affective or ideological proximity – or distance.

Bowlby hypothesized an 'anxious attachment' pattern as an indication of the constant anxiety experienced by children or adults when they establish interpersonal relationships, deriving from the insecurity of their very first relationships. The desire to receive love and attention may sometimes be masked by the casual rejection of close relationships involving emotional feelings. Such people form ambivalent relationships in order to avoid the possibility of a solid bond.

Over time, sight becomes a surrogate for touch, and the notion of proximity changes with the concept of visual space (Hall, 1966). The world of tactile sensation is connected to the visual world in a synesthetic picture that also includes olfactory functions.

Liberman *et al.* (1982) maintains that in patients he terms 'psychosomatic', the development of the concept of space does not occur in the usual way and results in pseudo-development. There is no notion of a stable space; that is, no notion of the existence of objects when they are not actually present in the surrounding space. They cannot distinguish between abstract representation and immediate sensory data.

The types of behaviour exhibited may include the tendency to immediately break off and abandon relationships, alternated with attempts to come closer and form adhesive bonds. This is the result of the aforementioned difficulty of the Ego to construct space and maintain distance, and may well be connected to the patient's skin (Anzieu, 1974; Tustin, 1981).

Ulnik (2007) describes patients with skin diseases who may present a friendly attitude and then rapidly disconnect with no consideration for the other. This type of behaviour could be connected to an attachment figure that did not provide a safe affective base, but rather created the opposite. The absence of the emotional security that normally allows for separation is thus experienced as the threat of abandonment. When separation cannot be imagined as an integral part of the evolution of an attachment relationship, there will be a tendency towards symbiosis. The compulsive need to devote oneself to others may hide a need for attachment as well as an implicit resentment for the lack of emotional security experienced in childhood.

It is interesting to bear in mind that, in Bowlby's view, the basic evolutionary function of attachment is to create an inter-subjective environment that provides a baby with sensitive nurturing, and later evolves into an understanding of the nature of mental states.

1.6 The reflective function, or mentalization

This concept already existed in the Freudian notion of bonding, and referred to the qualitative transition from a physical connection to one of a more psychological nature. Fonagy and other authors developed this concept further, adding the notion of the reflective function of attachment.

Fonagy (in Fonagy *et al.*, 1991, 1995; Fonagy and Target, 1998; Fonagy and Bateman, 2006) believes that the first relational environment is important not only because it shapes subsequent relationships, but also because it provides the child with a processing system that will enable him to create mental representations of relationships. The psychological Self of the child is formed through the perception of being an individual who thinks and feels; this perception initially derives from being acknowledged and present in the mind of another person.

In the mother–child relationship, physical discomfort is felt and then dealt with by the mother. Through concrete actions, she shows the child that he is understood and that she experiences his discomfort as being undesirable – that is, the discomfort is reflected in the mother, and this leads her to act upon it.

Following this line of thought, Ammaniti (1999) stresses that mentalization is the ability to see both oneself and others in terms of feelings, beliefs, intentions and desires, and to think about one's own and others' behaviour through a process called 'reflection'. This capacity for reflective enactment helps the individual experience life as having meaning.

For example, one patient thought she understood the feelings of others, but her 'understanding' was achieved mainly by pathological projective identification: she was unable to consider the diversity of others and the reality of the interpersonal space.

1.7 Distance in space and affective distance

Anthropologist Edward T. Hall (1951, 1966) studied how adults perceive the concept of space in terms of distance. The primitive behaviour of attachment requiring close contact is a form of protection; distance then denotes rejection. Every individual has a personal system that determines the appropriate distance to keep between him or herself and others. This consists in many factors, including childhood and adult experiences of direct contact, issues of self-esteem and individual strategies developed to manage close contact with others.

If the child's initial experience of space occurs through tactile proximity, as he begins to walk he develops a concept of distance that is measured starting from his own body.

An affective mother–child relationship fosters the gradual development of an *affective distance*. The concept of internal and external space, both physical and mental, develops over time. The first interior space is the mouth, which represents a space both of union and of frustration. Tactile space is subsequently organized as the baby begins to perceive the limits of his or her body and the distance from others. The 'non-space' represented by what is initially a fusional relationship gradually diminishes, and new spaces emerge – for example, through the action of seeing and walking; thus notions of perspective and reversibility in a three-dimensional world begin to develop.

Acquiring visual space and spatial images makes permanent representations possible: these are not lost like the tactile experiences resulting from close physical contact.

In the beginning, the baby is unable to distinguish his own representation of the object from the object itself, and the person who looks after him from a concrete object. 'The notion of the absent object is an evolutionary process and is the precondition for creating symbols' (Liberman *et al.*, 1982, p. 351).

Hall distinguished different types of distance, each with its own set of circumstances and measurements (intimate, personal, social and public). These types of distance are defined in measurable terms of space and volume of the voices used in various situations. The distance between oneself and the other depends on the perception of the senses and the development of one's own sense of Self.

The acceptable distance to be kept between oneself and the other depends on many personal and social factors, starting from the 'acceptable' distance of bodies in specific situations. For example, in the animal world, distance is monitored by recognizing danger and possible escape routes; the distance a soldier keeps from the enemy is regulated by the possibility of reaching for a weapon.

The closest possible proximity between two human beings is experienced through sexuality or certain forms of physical activity, such as wrestling. In these cases, physical contact prevails and the predominant senses are tactile and olfactory. These situations are different from other types of intimate proximity, such as being in a crowded underground, where feelings and intentionality are different.

If someone feels too weak and dependent on someone else, they will want to reduce distance to a minimum. In the case of symbiosis, there is no distance: separation becomes equivalent to disintegration.

Although in psychoanalysis one can speak of an affective distance, this is a conception of space that is neither perceptible nor measurable. It is in fact a wider representation of space in which the qualities of the object are not only measurable in space and time (i.e. proximity, distance, temporal and spatial mobility), but also contain a psychic element that comes from ordinary vicissitudes of emotional development (Liberman *et al.*, 1982, p. 354). Affective distance is thus the result of two different types of distance, namely, physical and emotional. This includes one's own representation of body image, the limits and boundaries represented by the skin, and the type of relationship with the object.

Tustin (1981) claims that the absence of symbolization results in intrusive projective identification, whereby the Self protects itself inside the other. In the constitution of autistic nuclei, the role of the skin can be seen as a sort of 'Ego-sieve' and 'Ego-shell'. These are clinical manifestations of the failure of symbolization of the body and the skin. This might be the consequence of the use of either projective adhesion or mimetic identification.

1.8 The skin and the process of symbolization: the journey from sensory-dominated experience to symbolization

In a child's development, the process of symbolization develops through the acquisition of language when a symbol can be used to represent the object it symbolizes in its absence, and is experienced as being separate from the object (Jones, 1923; Winnicott, 1945; Segal, 1950; Freud and Rieff, 1963; Klein, 1980).

The importance of concreteness and visibility is particularly evident in the absence of mental representations of an internalized human object; this is the case of a defective development of the process of symbolization.

As already illustrated, the primitive experience of the skin is involved in the acquisition of the concepts of proximity or distance, starting from a physical and spatial conception and moving towards an affective one. The lack of symbolization of sensory experience means that the individual lives in a world of outward appearance; not only are they not aware of this, but they may come to consider themselves exceptionally adept in the art of profound relationships.

Here, the object-relation seems to have been experienced only in terms of sensory contact experience, without having undergone a transformation into complex thoughts and feelings. So when thinking of either people or objects, all that takes place is an evaluation of the surface. Choices then depend only on what one can touch, see and control by sight. One might say that some patients' lives have been guided by needs dictated prevalently by the senses or the body, which have never turned into real emotional needs of the Self.

The symbolization process marks the transition from the autistic and paranoid-schizoid mode of sensory experience that characterizes the first few months of life towards depressive functioning. If this transition does not take place, the autistic-like experience, which is predominantly sensation-dominated, remains as a sort of sediment at the base of the unconscious personality, devoid of symbolic transformation and unknown to the other more evolved side of the Self.

In the early stages of a child's development, the child does not need symbols. It is only during the process of separation that symbols appear, as the subject finds a symbolic way of interpreting his own perceptions of loss. The moment the child perceives his mother as an object, he acknowledges that she can comfort him and feel discomfort, just as he does. What develops is the perception of the other's point of view, the ability to experience guilt, mourning, empathy and atonement.

What gradually emerges is the recognition of the Self as a subject that can give objects meaning and have an experience in the world accompanied by thoughts and personal feelings.

Winnicott (1953) conceives the potential space as the area that emerges between mother and child when the experience of unity is no longer sufficient or appropriate. The process of symbolization then can occur in different ways.

During the union with the mother, the baby does not perceive the mother as another person. He is at one with her and so he is not aware of his needs simply because these needs are completely satisfied without his having to act on them. The mother at this point is not visible as a separate subject. This separation between mother and child as two different beings occurs gradually, and early frustrations give rise to desires of reunification. In the intermediate space between mother and baby, three elements then arise: the symbol, the symbolized object and the subject who interprets it. Symbols do not arise without desires, and frustrations, when appropriately managed, help the process of separation.

In this potential space, the child begins to experience an inner and an outer reality, a Me and a non-Me, and an awareness of himself as subject who interprets this new experience. The child gradually begins to put together his own thoughts and feelings. During this first period of life, frustrations necessarily ensue and are met with empathy. If, however, separation is premature, if it is chronic or if the illusion of being a unit is interrupted abruptly by a major event, the baby dis-invests in the object, and this internal dialectic process may fail. The psychological dialectic between the two states of being together and being separate allows for the ability to generate personal meanings represented through symbols and mediated by individual idiosyncrasies.

Failure in this process may manifest itself in different ways. If there are problems in the process of separation (for example, if the baby has physical problems, or the mother has a personality disorder, or the surrounding environment is highly problematic), the child's defensive manoeuvres may be so extreme that any attempt to attribute meanings to objects fails. The original state of 'being one' is no longer satisfactory: differences are either not acknowledged or there is no need to attribute meaning to these differences. Since the baby is not adequately protected at this point in life, he experiences a general state of suffering that results not in psychological pain but in a state of non-experience (Ogden, 1980). Because of this withdrawal into a state of non-experience, perceptions and sensations remain unprocessed and no meaning is attributed to them, thus precluding any possibility of initiating a dialectical process (Meltzer, 1986; McDougall, 1989; Green, 1993; Grotstein, 1997).

If we consider real life as an experiment where one is required to move beyond a state of omnipotence, we can see how the problems described above can lead to imaginative failure. Imagination becomes tangible and gratifying, and replaces real life, which has become too disturbing. So the subject may not understand much about real life at all, since it lacks any meaning attached to what is experienced. Things are what they are (symbolic equation, Segal, 1957). The distinction between the symbol and what is symbolized collapses, leaving no space to debate ideas and feelings.

1.9 The concept of distance and the symbolization of space

The concepts of space and time emerge at the moment of separation. Original intelligence creates order out of disorder. Taking possession of space means leaving the autistic space and entering a menacing world.

It is the notion of the absent object that signals the development of the ability to create differentiated symbols. The qualities of proximity and distance in space, as well as the passing of time, will evolve in the external world in terms of sounds and places. This development follows an order that gradually evolves in parallel with the development of the interior psychic space, which forms through the ordinary vicissitudes of emotional development.

Tustin (1972) spoke of the functional deficits of an Ego that is unable to symbolize. Due to the mechanism of intrusive identification, these subjects live through the life of others, maintaining a defensive armour while also attempting to penetrate the armour of others.

I noticed that these patients were unable to endure separation and distance, even though, conversely, closeness triggered anger and anxiety. What emerged were distortions in the ideas of personal proximity and distance as well as in the relationship between the skin of the Self and the skin of the other.

The logic and paradox of opposites reveals the ways in which opposites are intertwined in the process of symbolization, and a third element can be added to the notions of *similar* and *opposite*: the emerging ability to discern the more subtle differences in experiences.

The child begins to experience time as well as space: in order to obtain what is needed from the object, the child introjects the idea of time, therefore establishing a relationship between space and time. The period of waiting requires the baby to develop a notion of time, which is vital for the child to tolerate change. When a patient begins to acquire the concept of time during the process of analysis, he or she can finally apply it to the analyst and the analytic situation, accepting that it takes time and active involvement to improve or get better.

During the phase of development, the child organizes other sensory spaces in addition to that of the skin: touching, hearing and feeling will be ways of becoming aware of the existence of other people and their senses. There is an immediate space near the baby's body that brings with it the notion of me and not-me: an experience of limits, of containment and of contact.

Notes

1 Non-represented states entail the concept of representation but are to be found at the very early stages of development.
2 Among these I would like to mention the works of: Aisenstein (1993, 2006); Anzieu-Premmereur (2009, 2010); Anzieu-Premmereur and Cornillot (2003); Botella and Botella (2001, 2005); Cassoria (2008, 2009, 2012); Civitarese (2008, 2013); Eshel (1998, 2013); Fenton et al. (2010); Grotstein (1986); Khan (1964); Levine (2012); Oliner (1988); Reiner (2012); Reed (2009); Scarfone (2011).
3 The term 'black holes' introduced in astrophysics in 1968 by J. Wheeler was later developed by scientific research and used in the field of science fiction. Black holes represent a series of events in the universe following the death of stars that collapse after reaching a certain stage of development. The stars that die have such a strong gaseous density and such a huge centripetal force that not even light can pass through them. Therefore, black holes represent areas of space-time that contain elements devoid of existence, which are not visible and can be identified from Earth only by the use of x-rays that pick up the gas surrounding them (Hawking,1993).

References

Aisenstein, M. (1993) 'Psychosomatic solution or somatic outcome: the man from Burma', *International Journal of Psychoanalysis*, 74, 371–382.
Aisenstein, M. (2006) 'The indissociable unity of psyche and soma: a view from Paris Psychosomatic School', *International Journal of Psychoanalysis*, 87, 667–680.
Ammaniti, M. (1999) 'Attaccamento e processo di mentalizzazione', *Psicologia clinica*, III, 1/1999.
Anzieu, D. (1974) 'Le moi-peau', *Nouvelle Revue de Psycanal*, 9, 195–208.
Anzieu-Premmereur, C. (2009) 'The dead father figure and the symbolisation process'. In L. Kalinic and S. Taylor (eds), *The dead father: a psychoanalytic inquiry* (pp. 133–144), New York: Routledge.
Anzieu-Premmereur, C. (2010) 'Fondements maternels de la vie psychique', 71st Congress of French-speaking analysts, *Bulletin de la Société Psychoanalitique de Paris*, 98, 193–238.
Anzieu-Premmereur, C. and Cornillot, M. (2003) *Pratiques psychoanalytiques avec les bébé*, Paris: Dunot.
Barrows, K. (2008) *Autism in childhood and autistic features in adults*, London: Karnac.
Bion, W. R. (1962) 'A theory of thinking'. In *Second thoughts: selected papers of psychoanalysis* (pp. 110–119), New York: Jason Aronson, 1967.
Bion, W. R. (1970) *Attention and interpretation*, London: Tavistock Publications.
Botella, C. and Botella, S. (2001) 'La figurabilité', Rapport au Congrès de Langue Française, Paris, *Revue Française de Psychanalyse*, 45(4).

Botella, C. and Botella, S. (2005) *The work of psychic figurability: mental states without representation*, London: Routledge.

Bowlby, J. (1986) *Vinculos afectivos. Formacion, desarrollo y perdida*, Madrid: Morata [*The making and breaking of affectional bonds*, London: Tavistock Publications, 1979].

Cassoria, R. M. (2008) 'The analyst's implicit alpha-function, trauma and enactment in the analysis of borderline patients', *International Journal of Psychoanalysis*, 89(1), 161–180.

Cassoria, R. M. (2009) 'Reflections on non-dreams-for-two, enactment and the analyst's implicit alpha-function'. In H. Levine and L. Brown (eds), *Growth and turbulence in the container/contained* (pp. 151–176), Hove, UK; New York: Brunner-Routledge.

Cassoria, R. M. (2012) 'What happens before and after acute enactment? An exercise in clinical validation and the broadening of hypothesis', *International Journal of Psychoanalysis*, 93, 53–80.

Civitarese, G. (2008) *The intimate room: theory and technique of the analytic field*, London: Routledge.

Civitarese, G. (2013) *The violence of emotions: Bion and post-Bionian psychoanalysis*, London: Routledge.

Edwards, J. (1994) 'On solid ground: the ongoing psychotherapeutic journey of an adolescent boy with autistic features', *Journal of Child Psychotherapy*, 20(1), 57–84.

Eshel, O. (1998) '"Black holes", deadness and existing analytically', *International Journal of Psychoanalysis*, 79, 1115–1130.

Eshel, O. (2013) 'Patient-analyst "withness": on analytic "presencing", passion and compassion in states of breakdown, despair and deadness', *Psychoanalytic Quarterly*, 82, 925–963.

Fenton, A. A., Lytton, W. W., Barry, J. M., Lenck-Santini, P., Zinyuk, L. E., Kubik, S., Bureš, J., Poucet, B, Muller, R. U. and Olypher, A. V. (2010) 'Attention-like modulation of hippocampus place cell discharge', *Journal of Neuroscience*, 30(13), 4613–4625.

Fonagy, P. and Bateman, W. (2006) *Mentalisation-based treatment for borderline personality disorder: a practical guide*, Oxford: Oxford University Press.

Fonagy, P. and Target, M. (1998) 'Mentalization and the changing aims of child psychoanalysis', *Psychoanalytic Dialogues*, 8(1), 87–114.

Fonagy, P., Leigh, T., Kennedy, R., Mattoon, G., Steele, H., Target, M., Steele, M. and Higgitt, A. (1995) 'Attachment, borderline states and the representation of emotions and cognitions in self and other'. In D. Cicchetti and S. S. Toth (eds), *Rochester symposium on developmental psychopathology: cognition and emotion*, vol. 6 (pp. 371–414), Rochester, NY: University of Rochester Press.

Fonagy, P., Steele, H. and Steel, M. (1991) 'Maternal representations of attachment during pregnancy predict organisation of infant-mother attachment of one year of age', *Child Development*, 62, 891–905.

Freud, S. (1913) *The interpretation of dreams*, third edition, translated by A. A. Brill, New York: The Macmillan Company.

Freud, S. and Rieff, P. (1963) *General psychological theory: papers on metapsychology*, New York: Collier Books.

Green, A. (1983a) *Narcissism de la vie et narcissism de mort*, Paris: Minuit.

Green, A. (1983b) *Life narcissism, death narcissism*, London: Free Association Books.

Green, A. (1986) *On private madness*, London: Karnac.

Green, A. (1993) *Le travail du negatif*, Paris: Editions du Minuit.

Green, A. (1997) 'The intuition on the negative in playing and reality', *International Journal of Psychoanalysis*, 78, 1071–1084.

Green, A. (1998) 'The primordial mind and the work on the negative', *International Journal of Psychoanalysis*, 79, 649–665. Read at the Centennial Celebration of Bion's birth, held in July 1997 in Turin.

Green, A. (2002) *Idées directrices pour une psychoanalyse contemporaine*, Paris: Presse Universitaires de France.

Green, A. and Kohon, G. (2005) *Love and its vicissitudes*, Hove, East Sussex: Routledge.

Grotstein, J. S. (1986) *Of things invisible to mortal sight: celebrating the work of James S. G. Grotstein*, London: Karnac.

Grotstein, J. S. (1987) 'Making the best of a bad deal: on Harold Boris' "Bion revisited"', *Contemporary Psychoanalysis*, 23(1), 60–76.

Grotstein, J. S. (1989) 'Some invariants in primitive emotional disorders'. In L. B. Boyer and P. L. Giovacchini (eds), *Master clinicians working through regression* (pp. 131–155), Northvale, NJ: Jason Aronson.

Grotstein, J. S. (1990a) 'The "black hole" as a basic psychotic experience: some newer psychoanalytic and neuroscience perspectives on psychosis', *Journal of the American Academy of Psychoanalysis*, 18(1), 29–46.

Grotstein, J. S. (1990b) 'Nothingness, meaninglessness, chaos and the "black hole" I', *Contemporary Psychoanalysis*, 26, 257–290.

Grotstein, J. S. (1990c) 'Nothingness, meaninglessness, chaos and the "black hole" II', *Contemporary Psychoanalysis*, 26, 377–407.

Grotstein, J. S. (1993) 'Towards the concept of transcendent position: reflection on some of "the unborns" in Bion's cogitation', *Journal of Melanie Klein and Objects Relations*, 11(2), 55–73.

Grotstein, J. S. (1997) 'The psychoanalytic fascination with the concept of the primitive. In S. Alhanati and K. Kostoulas (eds), *Primitive mental states, vol. 1: across the lifespan* (pp. 1–22), Northvale, NJ: Aronson.

Hall, E. T. (1951) *The silent language*, Garden City, NY: Doubleday.

Hall, E. T. (1966) In M. Kete Asante, Y. Miike and J. Yin (2008) *The global intercultural communication reader*, New York: Routledge.

Hawking, S. (1993) *Hawking on the big bang and black holes*, Singapore: World Scientific.

Jones, E. A. (1923) *Essays in applied psycho-analysis*, London: International Psycho-Analytical Press.

Khan, M. (1964) 'Ego distortion, cumulative trauma, and the role of reconstruction in the analytic situation', *International Journal of Psychoanalysis*, 45, 272–279.

Klein, S. (1980) 'Autistic phenomena in neurotic patients', *International Journal of Psychoanalysis*, 61, 395–401.

Liberman, D., Grassano de Piccolo, E., Neborak de Dimant, S., Pistimer de Cortinas, L. and Roitmann de Woscoboinik, P. (1982) *Del cuerpo al simbolo*, Buenos Aires: Kargieman.

Mancia, M. (2003) 'Dream actors in the theatre of memory', *International Journal of Psychoanalysis*, 84, 285–952.

McDougall, J. (1989) 'One body for two'. In *Theaters of the body* (pp. 140–161), London: Free Association Books.

Meltzer, D. (1986) *Studies in extended metapsychology*, London: Clunie Press for the Roland Harris Trust Library.
Mitrani, J. (1996) *A framework for the imaginary*, London: Karnac.
Mitrani, J. (2008) *A framework for the imaginary*, second edition, London: Karnac.
Ogden, T. H. (1980) 'On the nature of schizophrenic conflict', *International Journal of Psychoanalysis*, 61, 513–533.
Ogden, T. H. (1989) *The primitive edge of experience*, London: Karnac.
Oliner, M. (1988) 'Anal components in overeating'. In H. J. Schwartz (ed.), *Bulimia: psychoanalytic treatment and theory* (pp. 227–254), Nadison, CT: International Universities Press.
O'Shaughnessy, E. (1964) 'The absent object', *Journal of Child Psychotherapy*, 1(2), 34–43.
Reed, G. S. (2006) 'The reader's lack: commentary on Wilson', *Journal of the American Psychoanalytic Association*, 54(2), 447–456.
Reed, G. S. (2009) 'An empty mirror: reflections on non-representation'. In H. B. Levine, G. S. Reed and D. Scarfone (eds), *Unrepresented states and the construction of meaning: clinical and theoretical contributions* (pp. 18–41), London: Karnac.
Reiner, A. (2012) *Bion and being: passion and the creative mind*, London: Karnac.
Rosenfeld, H. (1979) 'Transference psychosis in the borderline patient'. In J. Le Boit and A. Capponi (eds), *Advances in psychotherapy of the borderline patient* (pp. 485–510), New York: Jason Aronson.
Rosenfeld, H. (1987) *Impasse and interpretation*, London and New York: Tavistock Publications.
Scarfone, D. (2011) 'Repetition: between presence and meaning', *Canadian Journal of Psychoanalysis*, 19(1), 70–86.
Segal, H. (1950) 'Some aspects of the analysis of a schizophrenic', *International Journal of Psychoanalysis*, 31, 268–278.
Segal, H. (1957) 'Notes on symbol formation', *International Journal of Psychoanalysis*, 38, 391–397.
Spitz, R. (1965) *The first year of life: a psychoanalytic study of normal and deviant development of object relations*, New York: International Universities Press.
Tremelloni, L. (2005) *Arctic spring: potential for growth in adults with psychosis and autism*, London: Karnac.
Tustin, F. (1972) *Autism and childhood psychosis*, London: Hogarth.
Tustin, F. (1981) *Autistic states in children*, London: Routledge & Kegan Paul.
Tustin, F. (1986) *Autistic barriers in neurotic patients*, London: Karnac.
Tustin, F. (1990) *The protective shell in children and adults*, London: Karnac Books.
Tustin, F. (1992) 'On psychogenic autism', *Psychoanalytic Inquiry*, 13, 34–41.
Ulnik, J. (2007) *Skin in psychoanalysis*, London: Karnac.
Winnicott, D. W. (1945) 'Primitive emotional development'. In *Through paediatrics to psycho-analysis* (pp. 145–156), New York: Basic Books, 1975.
Winnicott, D. W. (1953) 'Transitional objects and transitional phenomena: study of the first not-me possession', *International Journal of Psychoanalysis*, 34, 89–97.
Winnicott, D. W. (1960) 'Ego distortion in terms of true and false self'. In *The maturational processes and the facilitating environment: studies in the theory of emotional development* (pp. 140–152), London: Karnac.
Winnicott, D. W. (1971a) 'Playing: a theoretical statement'. In *Playing and reality* (pp. 38–52), New York: Basic Books.

Winnicott, D. W. (1971b) *Playing and reality*. London: Tavistock Publications.
Winnicott, D. W. (1971c) *The Piggle: an account of the psychoanalytic treatment of a little girl*, London: Hogarth Press.
Winnicott, D. W. (1974) 'Fear of breakdown', *International Review of Psycho-Analysis*, 1, 100–107.

Chapter 2

About skin

The skin as a surface of the body

2.1 The theme of the surface

The theme of the surfaces of objects or people is common throughout some of these patients' stories, causing unease in the analyst because of the absence of expressive communication relating to feelings and thoughts.

During the sessions, as I myself experienced a world of surfaces, I did not feel that I was with the 'person' of the patient. The description of his or her story in the sessions would focus mainly on people they knew and in particular their aesthetic features or possessions; there was never any mention of these people's feelings or mental characteristics.

These patients wanted to prove that this way of looking at superficial aspects was normal, as it represents how things are in the world around us. Of course, it must be said that in today's consumer society, the external aspects of surfaces and shapes do indeed prevail: television commercials are there to prove it. But I found that their interest in appearance and surfaces was basic, even extreme, and it affected the choices they made.

So I decided to think more about the subject of skin and surfaces.

The relationship between the skin and the development of the Self are thoroughly analysed by D. Rosenfeld (1975, 1984, 1985, 1986) and by J. Ulnik (2007). Rosenfeld extensively describes his work with psychotic patients who are addicted to drugs, sex or video games, and illustrates the relationships between what he calls 'skin diseases' and the lack of 'normal' conceptualization of the skin.

Ulnik also looks into the relationship between the skin and psychic development, offering many case descriptions to support this hypothesis.

2.2 Appearance and the skin

In a figurative sense, the term 'surface' is used to signify the external aspect, the appearance. People's appearance serves as a representation of the Self in social contexts, and its variations express internal variables.

Roberto Fernandez (1978) studied the relationship between skin and clothes. The first clothes that replaced the foetal vernix were animal fur; subsequently, these were replaced by woven materials and finally by various forms of fabric. The original purpose of clothes was to protect the human body and to keep people warm. Initially, clothes were quite basic. Later they became richer, and ornaments were added.

The desire for a permanent ideal and protective presence gives rise to a narcissistic investment in the fantasies about bodily products (such as faeces and urine, which are substances that come into contact with the body): thus they become narcissistic representations of the subject. These derivatives can be symbolically expressed through valuable golden ornaments, and other jewellery, that serve a protective function.

Thus a person who is prone to wearing objects of great value wears them, as it were, as self-protective armour when they encounter difficult situations that might threaten their identity. Clothes and ornaments such as masks make it impossible to see emotional changes, visible through the skin, which is the outer shield of the interior. In addition, certain clothes such as uniforms represent membership to social groups and are masks of the group, carrying great symbolic significance.

2.3 Skin and identity

David Rosenfeld (1988) explains how the idealization of clothes is equivalent to the idealization of the skin containing the body by commenting on Charles Perrault's Donkey Skin story (Perrault, 1921 [1697]).

In this story, the princess's mother dies and her father decides he will marry the princess herself. She agrees, but only on condition that he provide a series of ever more beautiful clothes – a sort of second skin – which she refuses one after the other until she asks her father to give her the skin of his donkey. This donkey was especially valuable because it produced stools of gold and made the kingdom wealthy. Reluctantly the father offers this skin to his daughter, but the princess, disguised in the donkey skin, flees with the help of a fairy. In the end, she meets a prince who falls in love with her and asks for her hand in marriage; only then does she abandon the donkey skin and regain her true identity.

David Rosenfeld offers different interpretations of this story, linking them to his patients affected with skin diseases and deficits in conceptualizing the skin.

He interprets the contents of the story by highlighting the following points: the relationship between skin and identity; the pathological way of processing the experience of loss and abandonment through the use of the clothes that represent the dead mother; and the pathological process of mourning by both father and daughter. He sees the idealization of clothes as equivalent to the idealization of the skin, a substitute for the mother's body. Clothing is akin to the skin, which represents the person. He also points out the difficult adjustment of space – as illustrated by the story's characters for whom boundaries are determined by the skin – as well as the importance of distances and the role of projective identification.

In terms of projective introjection, in the analysis of his dermatological patients, David Rosenfeld found the same sequence of situations as can be found in this story, including: feelings of abandonment, loneliness and loss, destruction and suffering subsequent to a separation; projection of these feelings onto the other with the development of 'parasite-host' or 'folie-à-deux' relationships. Among the common themes found here we have: 'helping' another and giving an impression of generosity while actually intruding into the other; the subsequent return of what had been projected onto the other in an aggressive form through an apparent form of help but which in fact contained destructive parts; and the continuous search for support.

Another similarity pointed out by Rosenfeld between the characters of the story and his patients is the transformation of distance in intimate proximity through the use of an illusory skin that represents the object and serves as a shell that protects from the feelings aroused by the object, including feelings related to abandoning and being abandoned. The same function of protection may also be represented by direct aggression towards the Self, felt as a form of support, or by overactive or excessive muscle development (Bick, 1968).

An example of the reaction in the face of feelings of abandonment concerns one of my patients and what emerged following the cancellation of a session due to my absence. To avoid feelings of abandonment, the patient immediately decided to find a superfluous reason to avoid his daily duties. By identifying with the abandoning object, he was able to avoid feelings of disappointment, anger and sadness; furthermore, by imitating the analyst he has also demonstrated his appreciation and acceptance of the analyst as a model.

The relationship between the skin and problems of identity also emerge in the form of tattoos. In the past, certain prisoners or sailors inscribed tattoos in the skin as a sign of belonging to a group or as a sign of an identity in the absence of any symbolic feeling of their own identity.

In other cases, tattoos are used to fix the names of meaningful people in order to remember them and secure the relationship. In these cases, the names of loved ones are inscribed on the skin in order not to feel pain in the case of absence. Subsequently, when a conflict arises with the real person, the feelings of suffering can be transferred to the skin. Guillot and Cruz (1972) describe a case of a man who came out of prison and became aware of a serious betrayal by the beloved woman whose name was inscribed on his skin. He then wanted to tear this previously beloved name away; the tattoo remained as 'an irritating record on the skin' that he tried to eliminate at all costs by tearing at it.

2.4 The skin and the image of the body in autism

In the clinical case that will be discussed in Chapter 5 ('Sara: living on the surface'), the skin became the focal point when she began to experience a crisis of disintegration, during which she no longer seemed able to carry out a mental function of containment. The phantasy around the rupture of the abdominal skin with the subsequent spilling out of her internal organs terrified Sara and filled her with a fear of losing her identity. Her language expressed strange bodily sensations, which she attributed to individual organs: some had mental characteristics, like 'tired stomach', others were more physical, such as 'crushed liver' or 'frayed skin'.

This set of sensations, accompanied by feelings of terror, brings to mind the topic of body image and skin in autism, as described by Tustin (1986). This author describes the moments of terror that autistic children experience, and which are probably a result of a stream of sensations that cannot be controlled, similar to feeling excess internal liquid that threatens to overflow and spill out. These sensations terrify them with the thought of being sucked into a vacuum, towards a state of 'non existence', of not being, or of having a hole inside the body. Due to these sensations, the child with autism feels insecure within himself, and so he creates the illusion of building a tough exterior protection. It becomes necessary for the child to keep constant control of the situation in order to prevent this dangerous spillage: this hinders his or her ability to establish relationships with others.

Tustin (1986) asserts that, in the absence of adequate containment, the child will construct a protective autistic armour to defend himself against the terror of falling into a vacuum, of disintegrating and also losing a part of his body. This self-containment achieved via the skin is felt to guarantee continuity over time.

If containment is not good enough, these primitive states of terror can lead to the formation of a second skin (Bick, 1968) constructed by such children in order to hold themselves together; these states can also foster a mode of insensitivity, also used as a form of protection.

For these reasons, such patients require therapy based on close attention, human warmth and understanding in order to restore a reassuring cohesion and sense of continuity; at the same time, they need determination and firmness so that over time they will acquire a stronger sense of Self and abandon their defensive armour.

The bodily sensations that terrorized Sara during her crisis were related not only to her skin but also to her digestive system. These can be difficult for a patient to describe, since they belong to a pre-verbal period and therefore have no suitable words to represent them. These primitive states of bodily sensations are important in the development of body image and sense of Self. Children with autism seem to have an elementary image of the body as being made up of a system of tubes containing bodily fluids, held together by the skin (Rosenfeld, 1984; Tustin, 1986). During Sara's crisis, she reported that she felt her intestine as a single open tube; this led me to hypothesize she had experienced problems in relation to a containing, nourishing object that led to a terror of dying.

2.5 The skin suffers

In some cases, physical symptoms regarding the skin are manifested through eczema and allergic skin and mucosal reactions. Psychosomatic disorders can be thought of as turning to the body as an alternative to having to acknowledge and process early childhood experiences.

We know that during infancy the experience of separation initially occurs at the level of the skin.

Many psychoanalysts have taken an interest in the problems of eczema and allergies. Marty *et al.* (1963) and McDougall (1989) maintain that patients who are allergic, just like most patients with somatic disorders, have suffered disorders in relationships very early on in life.

Marty speaks of 'relationships with allergic objects' referring to particular object relationships in subjects that simply select the nearest possible object they can merge with: the subject tends to attract the other, then manipulate him or her in order to keep them close. This causes confusion between subject and object and blurs the boundaries between the two, leading to uninterrupted interpenetration and continuous use of projection and identification.

Canteros (1981) draws a connection between hypersensitive allergic reactions and the disproportionate response in defence of an identity that cannot be asserted. This kind of identity is likely of a syncretic or symbiotic kind, based on the notion of 'us', and is very difficult to convert into an individual identity.

Winnicott (1965) also attributes the development of allergic disorders to the child's difficulty in abandoning the state of fusion with the mother. Spitz (1965) maintains that skin diseases in infants emerge as a response to conflicting signals, through the withdrawal into the body, when the infant's affective need of being touched is not sufficiently met.

Sami-Ali (1991) claims that the origin of all allergic reactions is connected with the origin of subjectivity. The experience of any relationship begins by touching the other's skin; in the case of allergies, there is confusion around whether the active and passive positions of touching or being touched are equivalent. According to Sami-Ali, the allergic patient assumes that everything will be identical to their identity and will coincide perfectly with their needs. Their crisis erupts when the other reveals their 'otherness' by 'tearing themselves away' (reported by Ulnik, 2007, p. 87).

When patients with dermatological ailments face situations of traumatic loss or separation, they try to calm themselves through itching and scratching: they are creating an inflammation of the skin in order to deny their profound need for intimate contact (Pichon-Rivière, 1971, see eczema).

Itching then stimulates the need to scratch, which is associated with feelings of pleasure, but also with the need for more and more scratching. The itching–scratching cycle produces a certain degree of pleasure, which can be compared to sexual excitement.

According to Schur (1955), itching is connected to unconscious insights in the presence of danger. The somatic flood of fear is thus represented externally by itching.

As will be described in more detail in Chapter 5, Sara's eye-itching, which would emerge in a kind of paroxysm at the beginning of our sessions, replaced the mental representation of her irritation at having to accept a situation of dependence, even before I had begun to speak. The act of rubbing her eyes had the clear intention of making me think that our closeness was disturbing to her.

Anzieu (1987a, 1987b) says that, in the language of the skin, skin irritation is an undifferentiated element of psychological irritation or mental suffering.

2.6 The function of the skin

As described in the previous chapter, the skin is the first place of exchange and allows the development of the notions of both differentiation and union. It marks the boundaries between one and the other, starting from the external boundary of each.

If we consider the skin as the surface of the body, we can see it as a continuum that turns into the mucous membranes, corresponding with the various orifices. The skin has many functions and constitutes both a coating and a bearing for things beyond itself. It demarks individuality; it is the site in which non-verbal memories are inscribed; it can either represent a protective barrier or, on the contrary, it can be the entry point for diseases, through either contact or infection.

The unconscious mental representation of the skin is linked to the function of containment and the conservation of protective warmth, so it is related to sensory experiences and to a primitive image of the body.

The skin is intimately connected with emotions, demonstrating the influence of the mind over the body. Even Freud (1905a, 1905b) pointed out that emotions are expressed through the skin: fear causes goose bumps, embarrassment causes blushing, etc. In his study, he refers to the skin playing a role both in child sexuality and in hysteria. He viewed the skin as an extensive erogenous area, providing an erotic contact point, and held that the unconscious, unlike the conscious mind, has a significant impact upon somatic processes. He talked of the skin as providing an element of 'sameness' during the initial forms of the child's identification; in other words, 'being in another's skin', meaning that identification was a form of contact, and contact was a form of identification.

The skin thus serves the primitive function of containing parts of the Self, and constitutes an outer boundary. If the introjection of an object able to serve the function of containment does not take place in the early stages of life, the concept of interior space does not develop and the identity of the person may be confused. The identification with the object helps the process of integration and gives rise to the phantasy of an external and internal space.

In his unpublished presentation 'The skin as an organ of expression', Fernandez (1978) considers that humans beings need a large outer active surface, needed for metabolism that works from the inside outwards, and from the outside inwards; it is a structure of perceptions capable of recording what comes from the outside world. The skin thus is seen as a twofold sensory organ.

Anzieu (1987a, 1987b, 1995) argues that the skin plays a vital role in the development of the psychic apparatus, being a basis that allows the transformation of physical experiences towards the area of mentalization and thinking. For example, the tactile sense is of fundamental importance, even though it must ultimately give way when the time is right to the process of symbolization. Through physical stimuli, the skin helps the psychic apparatus form representations that constitute the Ego. According to Anzieu, the Ego-skin grows and allows the Ego to perform functions such as reception, perception, cohesion, support, protection, integration of the senses, identity and energy. The Ego-skin thus leads to the thinking-Ego. If primitive bodily experiences cannot be transformed and integrated through symbolization, the Ego will lose important functions.

If we consider that the skin has an inner layer that sends signals from within the child's body as well as an outer face that receives messages coming from the mother (i.e. the maternal environment) towards the child, we can see how this interface may initially create fantasies in the child of sharing her skin with the mother who looks after her. Over-stimulation of the skin from the outside environment can lead to narcissistic reinforcement, with a developing sense of a common 'invulnerable skin'. Conversely, if the external stimuli are too weak and hardly perceptible, the child may form a phantasy of a skin common to both mother and child, which is weak or full of suffering. This may lead to the development of masochistic features within the personality.

If differentiation and separation between the two interfaces happens too abruptly or completely, without any agency on the part of the child, what prevails may be phantasies that this common skin has been torn away and destroyed.

The normal development of the child, in the sense of having personal autonomy, happens with the disappearance of this phantasy of having a common skin with the mother. But if this phantasy remains, the separation process will be felt as a dangerous attack, leaving a wound in the child's sense of integrity.

The skin, then, is experienced as a containing object. Failure in the development of this primitive function due to an inadequate real object, or to phantasies of attacking the real object, makes introjection difficult. Bick (1968) proposed the term 'second skin' to indicate a particular situation of the infant who maintains a mental image of an unsatisfactory object. In such cases, real dependence will be replaced by a pseudo-independence, which aims to create a substitute containing 'skin'.

Anzieu (1987a, 1987b) extends this concept of 'second skin' describing different solutions to this failure, such as the formation of an autistic armour, the development of masochistic traits, a kind of muscle stiffness, or finally a tendency towards psychomotor agitation visible in both body and mind.

Anzieu illustrates the parallels between different functions of the skin and the corresponding Ego functions, starting with a basic concept of the relationship between organic and psychic elements. He describes nine main functions of the Ego-skin. If the child does not meet with a favourable maternal environment, the failure of each of these functions will give rise to specific symptoms that we find in adult patients who have difficulties in symbolization.

I would like to discuss here some features that may not have been sufficiently tested in Sara's case, but can nevertheless be connected to the symptoms she presented. Through the sensations of the skin, the child feels secure in the supporting arms and mind of the mother, beyond the support of the body in a physical sense. Conversely, the absence of an introjected supporting object may give rise to anxiety, experienced as emptiness (see Chapter 5).

The maternal care of the child's bodily functions (i.e. handling) defines the phantasy of an envelope-container containing the internal organs. The failure of this function will cause generalized, unexplainable anxiety, which cannot be soothed. In addition, the experience will be that of having an internal vacuum and holes in the internal organs (see Chapter 5, 'Sara: living on the surface').

The outer-most layer of the skin is a protective shield against external stimuli (anti-excitement). If there is a deficit in this protective function, the individual may develop Tustin's 'shell' type personality designed to protect a fragile Ego, or acquire defenceless paranoid anxieties. The protective shield against stimuli provided by the skin is replaced by formations such as Bick's aforementioned 'second skin'. The skin also has the function of individuation, in that it gives the sense of being a unique one and only. This bodily sense of being 'one' depends on how strongly the person feels their personal boundaries. If this function is not present, the person will feel a sense of alienation and lack of separation from the outside world. This may result in pathological projective identification (see Chapter 6, 'Irene: from robot-like to person').

Inter-sensorial functions give rise to what we call 'common sense'. This provides the function of integration and interconnection between the various feelings that come from the different experiences of the skin. A lack of such integration can determine the sense of a fragmented body, and the anarchic function of various organs (see Chapter 5, 'Sara: living on the surface'). For example, the function of sight becomes disconnected from the function of 'thinking'.

As I have said earlier, the skin has always been considered the area par excellence of erotogenic experience (Freud, 1905a); spread all over the body, it gives way to the development of areas that become privileged for sexual functions. If the skin receives care on a purely narcissistic and libidinal level, it loses its ability to receive and produce pleasure authentically, becoming a mere surface that carries a sense of invulnerability or immortality.

The over-sexualization of the skin and the mucous membrane, detached from the world of feelings, demonstrates a defect in the process of symbolizing the concept of skin, as if affective exchanges were merely relegated to the sensations coming from the skin and the mucous membrane, rather than having more profound meaning. Repeated sensory experiences in this mode substitute the concept of the passing of time: they exist in a timeless zone.

In the infant's state of complete helplessness, she looks for an object that can offer contentment and contain parts of the Self; this could be in the form of a sound, a voice, a sort of support.

In addition to the skin sensations, the Ego is also formed by visual sensations: the child must have an overall picture of himself in order to perceive his unity. If the other looks at you, then you exist. In cases of fragmentation of the Ego, to restore the sense of identity, it becomes necessary to attract the gaze of the other. This then leads to an identification with the image that the other gives you. It is important not only to be caressed, but also to be seen.

One of my psychotic patients, Ambra (Tremelloni, 2005), had a very confused identity and would change the colour of her contact lenses daily in order to change the colour of her eyes. When she came to the threshold of the consultation room, she wanted to make sure I recognized her, since the change in the colour of her eyes, in her own mind, gave her a totally different look. The outer surface of things had great importance to her in terms of her identity, and she imagined these outer surfaces as being the only elements that characterized a person.

Ogden (1992), defining a primitive way to gain experience in the 'autistic-contiguous' mode, declares that the experience of the skin surface is vital. It represents the point of convergence between the infant's idiosyncratic proto-symbolic world of sensory impressions and the interpersonal world, made up of objects that are separated from the infant and out of his omnipotent control.

In the early days of life, the child begins to develop feelings in his relationship with the world as it is introduced to him by the mother. Bodily care of the child passes through the skin into the 'inner' world, creating the experience of rhythm, periodicity, sequences, and giving an embryonic idea of time. The child may also develop a sensory-dominated way of being, perhaps better described as 'non-being', isolating his potential Self from all that is outside of this sensory-dominated world.

There are two functions of the skin that are equivalent to maternal functions: protection and acknowledgement. Skin disorders may express the traumatic loss of a narcissistic protective function. The absence of a protective object that can acknowledge the subject poses as an obstacle to the vital initial symbiosis. This absence remains in the mind as a longing for contact or fusion.

If the acknowledgement is not internalized, patterns of rejection may emerge, leading to feelings of 'strangeness' and of not being able to establish a proper sense of belonging (see Chapter 6, 'Irene: from robot-like to person').

In short, at a very primitive stage, parts of the personality are held together by the skin, which acts as the outer boundary. The skin serves then to contain parts of the Self. This function is dependent on the introjection of an external object that is capable of containing. If this function is not introjected, the concept of interior space cannot develop, and if the object is not introjected into the interior space, the identity of the person will be confused. When identification with the object does take place, it replaces the integration of the primitive state and gives rise to the phantasy of an inner and outer dimension.

2.7 Autism and the skin

In her study of autism in children, Tustin (1972) stressed the importance of the child's first sensory impressions and the creation of the personal world of sensations in which he lives. This world constitutes a system of primitive survival, a way to generate a primitive sense of identity that prevents the child from feeling that he is disappearing. It is through the skin that the first experiences of contact with the outside world begin to be differentiated into sensations of softness and comfort, and those of harshness.

Ogden (1992) highlights that the experience of the skin surface is very important because it constitutes the point of convergence between the world of proto-symbolic sensory impressions, which are idiosyncratic to the child, and the interpersonal world, which is made up of objects that are separated from the baby and thus out of his omnipotent control.

The new-born emerges in a state of total weakness; he searches for an object that can support parts of the Self, such as physical contact, a sound or a voice. Alvarez (2012) notes that the skin is not the only element that serves the containing function; there may be other elements that facilitate the integration of the child, such as the mother's constant attention and contact over time, her strong support for his body, and eye contact.

In thinking about these concepts in terms of my analytic work, I realized that, with patients whose symptoms were the result of a serious lack of primitive containment, I would frequently and spontaneously recall details of recent sessions in a more regular way than I would with other more integrated patients. I concluded that these thoughts, at an unconscious level, offered the support these patients needed. I felt I had to constantly hold them in my mind, long after the sessions. I often also felt the need to discuss their cases with others. This mental activity of supporting in my mind could be explained at a conscious level as being my particular concern for the development of the analytic work with that particular patient. At a deeper level, however, this mental support actually produced greater continuity and stability in the patient's own mind: at an unconscious level, the patient would feel thought about in a more continuous way.

I would now like to illustrate the concepts of Bick, Meltzer and Liberman regarding the primitive processes of identification and the role of the skin.

2.8 Meltzer's 'two-dimensional world'

In considering the meaning of surfaces, Meltzer (1974) describes a two-dimensional way of mental functioning apparent in certain types of autism, in which the internal space does not exist. Only the surfaces of the Self and the objects are experienced, and the meaning of objects is inseparable from the sensory qualities that are perceived from the surface (see Part III).

Even the Self is experienced as a surface with no inner space. In this two-dimensional situation, the object cannot be internalized or thought about because there is no mind capable of such fantasies, thoughts and memories. The object is perceived only in the sensory qualities of its surface. There is no awareness of an internal space, and only tactile and visual perceptions are considered important. In this case, identification can only happen at an adhesive level.

2.9 Adhesive identification

The concept of adhesive identification has been described by Bick (1968) and Meltzer (1974) to indicate a type of identification in the most primitive stages of life, when projective identification fails in the absence of an internal space where experiences can be projected. A defect in the development of the sense of internal space thus determines a tendency to interact with objects in a two-dimensional way.

When the mother holds the infant, he will react quickly in response to the sensations felt from the skin: this contact facilitates the process of joining and adhering to the mother and restores the feeling of being united with her. These sensations give the child a sense of safety and continuity of the body.

In the absence of such an exchange of affective communication, however, this adhesive mode of being will provide a solution that is necessary for survival, as in the case of autism. Adhesive identification is used in an attempt to create or restore a rudimentary sense of cohesion with the maternal surface. The surface of the other is used to substitute the lack of meaning in the relationship, which would develop for a child with a mother who is receptive to his needs.

As an example of this, in the analytic relationship some patients use adhesive identification as a way of coming into contact with me through my physical presence alone. They then fall into desolation and despair as soon as they leave my studio.

2.10 Mimetic introjective identification

Here I would also like to mention the concept of mimetic introjective identification as outlined by Liberman *et al.* (1982): this occurs in patients who lacked support early on in their development. Such children, who do not develop an awareness of an inner physical and emotional life, tend to possess a one-dimensional view of the Self – what one might call the 'façade image' – and feel the need to come into physical contact with this 'flat object', which is all that they know of the outside world. They try to establish an illusory union with the other by mimetically incorporating their superficial characteristics: they remain attached to the other's exterior, becoming part of the other, much like a stamp that becomes an integral part of the envelope it is attached to.

References

Alvarez A. (2012) *The thinking heart*, London and New York: Routledge.
Anzieu, D. (1987a) *El yo piel*, Madrid: Biblioteca Nueva.
Anzieu, D. (1987b) 'La concepcion del yo-piel', *Actualidad Psicologica*, 134, 11–13.
Anzieu, D. (1995) *The skin-ego*, London: Karnac Books.
Bick, E. (1968) 'The experience of the skin in early object-relations'. In A. Briggs (ed.), *Surviving space: papers on infant observation* (pp. 55–59), London: Karnac, Tavistock Clinic Series, 2002.

Canteros, N. (1981) 'Nuevos aportes al significado de la alergia', unpublished presentation to C. I. M. P., Buenos Aires.
Fernandez, R. (1978) 'La piel como organo de expression', unpublished presentation to C. I. M. P., Buenos Aires.
Freud, S. (1905a) 'Three essays on sexuality', *S. E.* 7, 125–245.
Freud, S. (1905b) 'Psychical (or mental) treatment', *S. E.* 7, 283–302.
Guillot, C. F. and Cruz, S. (1972) 'Tatuaje carcelario: experiencia in una prison bonaerense'. In J. Ulnik (ed.), *Skin in psychoanalysis*, London: Karnac, 2007.
Liberman, D., Grassano de Piccolo, E., Neborak de Dimant, S., Pistimer de Cortinas, L. and Roitmann de Woscoboinik, P. (1982) *Del cuerpo al simbolo*, Buenos Aires: Kargieman.
Marty, P., M'Uzan, M. and David, C. (1963) *L'investigation psychosomatique. Sept observations cliniques*, Paris: Presses Universitaires de France.
McDougall, J. (1989) 'One body for two'. In *Theaters of the body* (pp. 140–161), London: Free Association Books.
Meltzer, D. (1974) 'Adhesive identification'. In A. Hahn (ed.), *Sincerity and other works: collected papers of Donald Meltzer* (pp. 335–350), London: Karnac, 1994.
Ogden, T. H. (1992) *The primitive edge of experience*, London: Karnac.
Perrault, C. (1921 [1697]) *The fairy tales of Charles Perrault*, London: George Harrap.
Pichon-Rivière, E. (1971) 'Aspectos psicosomaticos de la dermatologia'. In J. Ulnik (ed.), *Skin in psychoanalysis*, London: Karnac, 2007.
Rosenfeld, D. (1975) 'Trastornos en la piel y el esquema corporal', *Revista de Psicoanalisis*, 32(2), 309–348.
Rosenfeld, D. (1984) 'Hypochondriasis, somatic delusion and body scheme in psychoanalytic practice', *International Journal of Psychoanalysis*, 65, 377–387.
Rosenfeld, D. (1985) 'Distorcions des actes', *Nouvelle Revue de Psychanalyse*, 30, 191–199.
Rosenfeld, D. (1986) 'Identification and the Nazi phenomenon', *International Journal of Psychoanalysis*, 67, 53–64.
Rosenfeld, D. (1988) *Psychoanalysis and groups: history and dialects*, London: Karnac Books.
Sami-Ali, M. (1991) *Pensar lo somatico. El imaginario y la patologia*, Buenos Aires: Paidos.
Schur, M. (1955) 'Comments on the metapsychology of somatization', *Psychosomatic Study of the Child*, 10, 119–164.
Spitz, R. (1965) *The first year of life: a psychoanalytic study of normal and deviant development of object relations*, New York: International Universities Press.
Tremelloni, L. (2005) *Arctic spring: potential for growth in adults with psychosis and autism*, London: Karnac.
Tustin, F. (1972) *Autism and childhood psychosis*, London: Hogarth.
Tustin, F. (1986) *Autistic barriers in neurotic patients*, London: Karnac.
Ulnik, J. (2007) *Skin in psychoanalysis*, London: Karnac.
Winnicott, D. W. (1965) *The maturational processes and the facilitating environment*, London: Hogarth.

Chapter 3

About sight and beauty

3.1 Primacy of sight in getting to know the outside world

In my work with patients with autistic traces, I have often been struck by the fact that the sessions mainly revolved around descriptions of the appearance of the surrounding world.

This consideration makes me think of my patient Irene (see Chapter 6) during the initial phases of analysis: when she started to catch glimpses of the possibility of emerging from her isolation, coming closer to others and looking for elements to introject that would enable her growth, she started to take part in group discussions with psychiatric patients in the hope that she might be helped to understand something about herself.

Apparently, at that time her paranoid preoccupations had decreased but she still lacked the ability to really listen in symbolic terms. What seemed strange to me was that her greatest preoccupation and anxiety derived more from her fear of getting lost or of not being able to find the building or the sign for the venue of the meeting, as opposed to feeling out of place or finding it difficult to participate in a group of unknown and problematic people.

The visual recognition of the environment became a reassuring element in a context of complex feelings and thoughts related to encountering other people. She could find reassurance only through what she could see with her own eyes.

Seeing is a sensory experience that gives immediate information about the outside world. In fact, beauty is immediately perceived by the eyes and the ears; this is the case, for example, when one listens to music. Sight and hearing are considered 'noble senses' because, unlike smell or taste, they are measurable and can therefore be translated through the intellect. It is said that 'something is evident' to mean that is it immediately clear and does not need reflection. But what I felt was missing in order to form an image of the patient's life were the real-life experiences of the narrating subject. Stating that perceived reality is beautiful or ugly merely gives an indisputable evaluation that does not stimulate any form of thought process.

Vision is an enigma formed by the union of the seer and the see-able. Seeing does not require thinking; it is a perception of the body.

When we speak of 'love at first sight', we want to highlight the power and the speed of the gaze. In this case, the dream of rediscovering a total, satisfying love, comparable to a primitive idealized object relation, comes true. Is this due to an instinctive identification and imitation of the other's physical manifestations? Can we consider this an immediate transferal relationship of infantile nature? Children react immediately when they encounter something new, displaying different emotions through facial expressions and physical behaviour. In adults, however, the immediate knowledge of the other through sight is processed over time by a thinking part, which may lead to partial disappointment with regards to primitive idealization.

In clinical practice, I found that love at first sight in some patients represents the discovery of an escape route from the analytic work, in that a gratifying relationship can be achieved quickly, unlike analytic thinking, which is lengthy and difficult. Love at first sight coincides with the lightning perception of the other person as a mirror image of oneself, the projection of one's emotional state and the discovery of some signs of similarity. It is the search for a narcissistic experience in which the subject falls in love with an 'idealized identical'. Getting to know something that is different – and then approaching it – involves a process of separating, acknowledging and tolerating differences, and pausing; in other words, taking a space in time to reflect on the information gathered through the senses.

Meltzer and Harris Williams (1988), in citing Hazlitt (1822) and Flaubert (1857), reflects on love (or hate) at first sight. He specifies that the original meeting of the eyes gives a first level of evident information and a second level of immediate emotions, that is, of passions, sympathy or antipathy. A third level is represented by feelings of suspicion, prejudice or aversion when faced with a stranger, especially in a non-formal situation where social masks are removed. This means that there is a fear of a certain level of vulnerability (hidden and often unacknowledged) in the encounter with the unknown other. Eye contact aims to get to know the person comprehensively and definitively.

With regards to the eye's function of seeing, the French philosopher Merleau-Ponty (1945) states that vision is accomplished not only through the eye's perception, but also from within the body: what determines vision is 'the essence of being'.

In his work 'Eye and mind', he states that we see not only the things the world is made of; we also see ourselves in the world. The body sees the surrounding world through the way it sees itself. This reflectivity results in the ambiguity of vision. The manifest visibility of things must be reconsidered in the body through a latent, secret visibility. Things that are visible to us have an internal equivalence in our body. When we see something, we feel its presence in a visceral way, which Merleau-Ponty called 'carnal formula'. Not only is there no distinction between the thing and our mental representation of it, but there is also no absolute distinction between the subject who sees and the object that is seen: the person who sees and the object being seen are cut from the same cloth and share a unity of being.

When Irene (see Chapter 6) could see no difference between the vitality of shop mannequins and that of living people, she expressed her unconscious state of mind in which life was confused with – and close to – that of death.

According to the French philosopher, one of the properties of the visible is that of having a double invisible: for example, when we look at a painting, it does not describe to us its true depth, but it appears to us through processes that have meaning for us, such as colour or perspective, and which allow our perception to reconstruct depth.

3.2 The meaning of surfaces and Meltzer's two-dimensionality

As I have previously stated, in listening to some of my patients' stories I noticed how interested they were in the details of the outward appearance of people, objects and environments: this raised questions about the focus they placed on exteriority, forms and surfaces, as opposed to the contents or meanings of events. What was perceived by sight took on definitive importance in the process of considering the outside world.

Ogden (1992) describes the sensory nature of the initial experience of contact with the outside world as an autistic-contiguous primitive experience that originates from the cutaneous surface. I think that the great interest in the surfaces of surrounding people and objects was linked to a primitive mode of getting to know the world, while the lack of symbolization and of an interior space had hindered the process of attributing personal meanings to perceived reality.

My initial questions about the predominant interest in surfaces reminded me of Meltzer's thought (1974), developed in his studies on autism. He applied the concept of dimensionality to mental functioning, in which the various dimensions of the object relationship represent stages of evolutionary development. The autistic world, in which the centre of the world is represented by the body itself, is considered as being one-dimensional. In this dimension, there is confusion between gratification and fusion with the object, and the events of the outside world happen around the Self and cannot be used for creative thinking or memory.

At a later stage, the world of the child with autism becomes two-dimensional, but there is still no idea of an internal space: there are only experiences of contact with one's own and the other's surfaces. The Self is experienced as a surface without an internal space. Meltzer (1974) says that the experience of objects is inseparable from the sensitive qualities that can be known only through surfaces. The mind is not capable of fantasies about the object, nor of thoughts and memory. For autistic children, the sensitive qualities of surfaces are the significant parts they tend to adhere to or lean on: in this phase children adhere to the superficial qualities of objects without considering them as separate.

In contrast, the three-dimensional position implicates the formation of an internal space within the containing object. The idea of the orifices of one's body starts to form, along with the idea of a containing space within both the object and the Self. The desire to be contained leads to the experience of containing. This establishes the possibility of passing feelings from one to the other, and activates the process of projective identification. When the Self and the object differentiate, the concept of space is formed.

In an individual's history, the return from a three-dimensional mode to a two-dimensional one is a defensive operation aimed at preventing the feeling of an interior space, perceived only as the seat of painful thoughts and feelings due to deadly objects that must be eliminated from the mind.

This explains the difficulty in transforming a predominantly sensory world into a symbolic world for those patients who have renounced an inner world that involved an unbearably painful experience.

A fourth dimension, according to Meltzer, is represented by time, which enriches the development of the Self and allows for the idea of a possible future. In patients with autistic mental states, there is no idea of the possibility of imagining one's future as different from the present or the past. This is particularly evident in the obsessive ideation in which it is impossible to move on from the past and the present. A sign of progression in analysis is the possibility of feeling that the conjugation of one's thoughts can give rise to a new life perspective.

Meltzer, following Bick's innovative ideas about skin, proposes the term adhesive identification to indicate an early attempt to create – or recreate as a defence – a rudimentary sense of one's own corporal cohesion through bodily sensory perceptions.

Bick (1968) described the primitive external object as 'a complex, undifferentiated object, composed of experiences of continuous interaction between physical and emotional holding, the mother's mental containment, and the bodily surface of the child'. The contact between the mouth and the nipple creates a primitive sense of a containing object, but if the mother does not have a good containing function, the child creates the phantasy of a skin that has a secondary containing function, thus replacing dependency with pseudo-dependency. Hence the notion of a 'second skin' with adhesive qualities.

In the two-dimensional object relationship, the object is perceived as an area that offers only sensory or sensual experiences. The feeling is the object. In analysis, the difficulty lies in supporting the patient to give up this mode of human relationships and enhance the value attributed to the feelings that pass between two people.

3.3 Interest in beauty

In some patients, the prevailing quality of what was being noted or appreciated in the description of people, characters in dreams, objects or environments concerns the notion of beauty: these patients always try to surround themselves with beautiful people and things, and they dream of living in a world devoid of imperfections.

In his history of beauty, the Italian philosopher Umberto Eco (2004) describes how over the centuries the concept of beauty has changed in relation to the object being considered – for example, art or nature – or in relation to the evaluation criterion depending on the historical period and cultural development of the time.

In certain periods, the concept of beauty has been linked to the concept of good. When we find that something is beautiful or graceful, we express something that we like and that we want for ourselves. In this sense, beauty represents what is desired, in the same way that something good, that we like, is desired. The concept of good could also be related to an ideal: we can admire a heroic action performed by another person and judge it to be good or beautiful, but this does not necessarily lead us to wish to reproduce it. In this case, what is good is not desired.

The evaluation of beauty can also contain a desire to possess, linked to feelings of envy, greed and jealousy. But the enjoyment of beauty has nothing to do with the desire to possess: a fresco by Giotto or Mozart's music bring us spiritual enjoyment, with particular intensity for each, limited in time, completely independent of the notion of possession.

The problem is that when the object that is loved and desired is no longer present, it causes suffering. In this sense, the need to see everything as beautiful excludes a link between the enjoyment that comes from sight and the experience of suffering, which concerns the realm of feelings.

These patients have a diffused vision of beauty that does not seem to belong to a search for an authentic aesthetic experience. In aesthetic philosophy, we speak of aesthetic experience to indicate a unique ability to find spiritual significance in material experiences. This is what one can experience before the beauty of certain works of art. Beauty thus becomes the fruit of a 'relationship' between the artistic object and the person that perceives it with his own individual sensibility.

I had many questions about what the category of 'beautiful' or 'beauty' was because they repetitively came to represent these patients' preferences in their vision of reality and of the relational space.

I wondered if the word 'beautiful', which was fundamentally vague and indeterminate, was being used as a 'thing in itself', not yet subjected to symbolization. As for the objects or the materials they were made of, beauty was often associated with brilliance, twinkling, bright colours: the material's exciting and attractive qualities.

I also wondered if the search for beauty was more akin to an adaptation to external formal or social models, in other words, to a trend, or if it was actually a form of reassurance connected to an archaic, indecipherable or persecutory world. Was this a pervasive, vague or generic need, or was it an expression of their adherence to a social group's view of the world that values appearances?

The perception of beauty was related to the external appearance of people, things and the material of which they were made. Was this part of the phenomenon of widespread aestheticization that currently characterizes the realms of media, television and advertising?

It is widely thought that success in life is attributed to the appearance of the body. Moreover, today in Italy we talk about 'ragazze imagine' (image girls) to indicate an activity of young, beautiful and elegant women who are invited to entertain guests on the occasion of certain social events, as if they were decorative items, stripping them of any subjective meaning. The word 'image' corresponds to a particular visual representation, such as a photograph, but is connected with the verb 'to imagine', which is very subjective.

Does the search for beauty in people mean doing away with the emotional complications of coming into contact with another person the way they are? Is beauty sought in the other an element that, by definition, is immune from the danger of rejection? Is it a model with fixed parameters or is it a way to see the world without variations or defects? Is this preconception essential in establishing human contact? Is this due to the fact that it is impossible to grasp the ambiguity of feelings in the encounter with the other? Does it imply reducing the other to anatomical peculiarities and standard physical forms?

Is seeking beauty everywhere a form of narcissistic mirroring, in which one's own beauty is projected onto another person? Or is it related to the need to be seen, observed and judged to be beautiful, as a consequence of the lack of recognition experienced in the earliest exchanges with the object? Is it a sign of escaping into mania in order to deny the suffering caused by a lack of contact?

I wondered if this need to limit beauty to the experience of encountering the world meant that the prevalence of primitive sensory experiences was reserved only to the organ of sight, with regards to the complexity of the emotional relationship. Had visual sensory perceptions dominated the representation of early childhood experiences?

All these questions were left unanswered and put on hold because the answers could only come by going deeper into the analytic work.

3.4 Beauty and the aesthetic conflict

Meltzer (in Meltzer and Harris Williams, 1988) hypothesizes that at birth the child learns about the existence of external beauty from the relationship with the mother, starting with the initial vital contact with the breast. This sense of aesthetic satisfaction will undergo transformations when the initial perception of the mother's beauty becomes ambiguous: the infant will soon realize that the maternal internal world is variable and also contains mental pain. Thus, the child forms the perception of the secret space of the mother's Self. This is the origin of Meltzer's aesthetic conflict: every individual's creative potential is born from the aesthetic conflict.

The reciprocity of the aesthetic impact, which takes place between child and mother as well as between mother and child, constitutes the initial emotional experience of coming into contact with the qualities and potential of the mother's Self, and with the birth of one's own Self.

Meltzer states that if the object is only partial (e.g. the mother's breast), it remains devoid of complexity – feelings and thoughts – and only keeps its formal and sensory characteristics.

What I perceived in the stories of some of my patients was their lack of personal intimacy, in the sense of aesthetic conflict: emotions, complex experiences, mental pain and the thoughts associated with it were missing, as well as an interest and curiosity regarding the internal object of the Self. Because of an excessive process of projective or adhesive identification, their interest was geared more towards the observation of others than the observation of their own inner world. Their lack of aesthetic conflict limited their potential to find personal meaning.

3.5 Meltzer's aesthetic reciprocity

Given the aesthetic impact the child has on the maternal reality that fully welcomes him into the world, Meltzer (in Meltzer and Harris Williams, 1988) emphasizes the importance of the aesthetic impact the child has on the mother or on the parents. Their imagination about his potential, along with their love, promotes the formation of the child's internal world, which will develop individually and give rise to his personality.

Likewise, in the analytic process, aesthetic reciprocity represents the analyst's interest in finding those mysterious aspects of inner beauty and potential within the patient. In this way, the analyst instils hope that the patient may be able to find a new internal structure, thus stimulating greater depth in self-analysis.

The defensive and complicated defences gradually erected during personality development prevent the person from enjoying the beauty of relationships. We can say that the experience of aesthetic reciprocity in analysis is confirmed over time when, after having overcome the inevitable clashes, misunderstandings and pain, one reaches a form of alliance, mutual understanding, admiration and trust.

3.6 Visible beauty or beauty of the bond?

Irene (see Chapter 6) was a beautiful young woman; nonetheless, she had a propensity towards ugliness in the sense that she neglected her body and her clothes and made no attempt to bring out her natural beauty. She also tended to surround herself with shabby people who were worn out and disorganized – both physically and psychologically. Despite the fact that her mental state and feelings of social inclusion improved during her analysis, this tendency was resistant to change as its roots lay in her personal history. In fact, her object relationship was characterized by a lack of interest and attention, by violence, neglect and poverty. The only possibility for her to look after herself, to put on make-up and dress up, was in 'make-believe' situations: plays in which she took part.

She herself was amazed when she received compliments as a result of these transformations.

Another case in which the lack of beauty was troubling for me was the vision of a particularly ugly patient-child who was referred to me for psychotherapy (Tremelloni, 1987).

Although I had been made aware of the dysmorphic nature of this patient and I knew his kind of pathology, the aesthetic impact was paralyzing: his features did not correspond to a pre-existing model in my mind, and he displayed an overall lack of harmony. He was neither a child nor an adult; I could not guess his age, and his voice had a low tone and a high volume, more like an adolescent than a child. His blue eyes were large and protruding, his mouth open with an under-bite. His hair was sparse and albino. His behaviour was unpredictable, he moved constantly.

My first impression was of terror and rejection, brought on by my fear that I would not be able to connect with a being for whom I had no mental category. His external form and bizarre behaviour distanced me from him and prevented me from instantly welcoming him and imagining any possible communication. The uncanny experience evokes something scary, along with a lack of meaning of the experience itself (Freud, 1925). Was it the fear of not knowing how to approach this different thing that threatened my own narcissistic homeostasis? Or was it just my distress at the lack of symmetry and harmony in the form of this face?

I wondered how the colleague who had made the referral, while being an expert in the field of autism, had any hope that a new psychotherapeutic relationship could bring any further developments, considering that the previous one had failed. So, my bewilderment was distanced and projected on the referrer.

Ernesto had been referred to me because he had problems attending classes at school: he was particularly rebellious with teachers, unable to learn to read and write and did not communicate with classmates. In the family, he went from moments of being withdrawn to aggressive outbursts targeted at himself and others. He spent his days collecting and obsessively dealing with glass and metal objects.

In our first session, Ernesto began jumping excitedly from the floor to the chairs and then to the table; I could not understand what thought was propelling him to do this. Perhaps with these changes of position he sought attention, an affirmation of his being, in contrast with his psychic parts, which were paralyzing our communication.

I immediately felt defensively withdrawn because of his aesthetic appearance; I was unable to communicate and felt helpless and frightened by the responsibility that I was about to take on. I was frightened and fantasized that I would not know how to communicate with someone from an unknown world. How could I accept something different from my personal model of the child-patient? Was it the lack of standard bodily forms that kept me from grasping the humanity in this being? Or was my bewilderment due to his challenging way of wiping out my presence with his provocative behaviour? I felt I was being confused with one of the autistic metal or glass objects that Ernesto collected. He did everything through his behaviour to discourage any form of relationship: was it a test of strength or his inability to believe that he could be accepted and loved?

The immediate sensory experiences that occur through sight (called 'at first sight') are crucial experiences of beauty or ugliness, of something pleasant or scary. Are they disconnected from the complex sphere of feelings and thoughts stirred by the encounter with another person?

Despite these crippling doubts, I continued to observe Ernesto, waiting to reflect and see how we could be together. To be able to welcome him as he was, I needed a summary of the elements of his personal history and his physical and emotional pain. Questions and reflections remained regarding my initial moving beyond and away from his aesthetic appearance. What aesthetic reciprocity did this child experience in that moment, and at birth?

An object in my study was of great importance in constructing the transitional object between us. It was a large colourful wooden Pinocchio, which served as a children's coat hanger. When Ernesto noticed it, he hugged him passionately, lay down on the floor with him and said, 'You are the dream of my fantasies, giant of the sea'. From that identification with a character that was made of wood, had a deformed nose and slender legs, and was the same height as him, Ernesto began a relationship of affection. The puppet represented the possibility for an element that originated from a plant to turn into a live child.

In that moment, he was the one showing me his need to be loved and his courage in manifesting affection for an unknown person.

His psychotherapy continued with the birth of a loving and productive relationship. Therapeutic medical surgery on various aspects of his body, his growth and the development of our relationship transformed, in my eyes, his monstrosity into an aesthetic form which had become familiar and which aroused my affection and interest. Thus, a relationship rich with affection, sensitivity, intelligence and humour was born. Ernesto's hour of therapy had become a space 'rich with vitality, freedom and emotional contact' for us both.

When his therapy came to an end, he left me a story he had made up, with drawings and a text in which he described the relationships between the characters using many swear words. But in the final dedication, 'To my dearest T.', he added to the conventional 'hugs and kisses' the words 'and many caresses', through which I felt his nostalgia for warm primitive contact and his gratitude for the closeness he had experienced in our relationship.

In the formulation of mental pain and pleasure, Bion (1959) considers that positive and negative emotional bonds – including desire and interest – are always present, and that pleasure and pain are inextricably linked. This conflict produces real change (as a consequence of learning from experience, and not learning from information given by others), and must then find a symbolic representation in language in order to allow the processing of thought through condensation, abstraction and the tools of sophisticated thought. Tolerating this conflict comes from the strength of the Ego and resides in the 'negative capability' (Keats, 1817) – that is, the ability to exist in uncertainty, mystery, doubt, without reaching after fact and reason.

References

Bick, E. (1968) 'The experience of the skin in early object-relations'. In A. Briggs (ed.), *Surviving space: papers on infant observation* (pp. 55–59), London: Karnac, Tavistock Clinic Series, 2002.

Bion, W. R. (1959) 'Attacks on linking'. In *Second thoughts: selected papers on psychoanalysis* (pp. 93–109), London: Heinemann, 1967.

Eco, U. (2004) *Storia della bellezza*, Milan: Bompiani.

Flaubert, G. (1857) *Madame Bovary*, Paris: Michel Lévy Frères.

Freud, S. (1925) 'Negation', *S. E.* 19, 235–239.

Hazlitt, W. (1822) 'Letters'. In C. H. Charles (ed.), *Love letters of great men and women*, London: Stanley Paul & Co, 1924.

Keats, J. (1817) 'Letter to George and Thomas Keats', 21 December. In *The selected poetry of Keats*, New York: Signet Classic, New American Library, 1966.

Meltzer, D. (1974) 'Adhesive identification'. In A. Hahn (ed.), *Sincerity and other works: collected papers of Donald Meltzer* (pp. 335–350), London: Karnac, 1994.

Meltzer, D. and Harris Williams, M. (1988) *The apprehension of beauty: the role of aesthetic conflict in development, art and violence*, London: Karnac.

Merleau-Ponty, M. (1945) *Le visible et l'invisible*, Paris: Gallimard, 1979.

Ogden, T. H. (1992) *The primitive edge of experience*, London: Karnac.

Tremelloni, L. (1987) 'The psychotherapeutic treatment of a psychotic child with marched autistic feature', *Psychoanalytic Psychotherapy*, 3 (1), 11–25.

Part II

Chapter 4

Clinical examples

4.1 The mask of the Ego

Groddeck (1929), a contemporary of Freud, was the founder of psychosomatic medicine. He employed the term 'mask' to define the use of the word 'I'. When we use the word 'I' to denote inner life when we communicate with others, we make a mistake. We refer to a Self, but this is something which is acquired over time: the 'I' takes on the function of a mask with regards to the subject's internal truth.

Language is connected with the problem of identity and thinking, and is therefore also connected to the deepest meaning of the Self. It expresses distortions created by an only partial understanding of the subject's own inner life. The word 'I' used as an expression of the individual Self with respect to the surrounding world could therefore be considered a false idea of individuality.

Primitive identification occurs with the 'It' (in German, *Es*) from which the first sense of Self evolves. The 'I' is a Self, which is created later, as opposed to that first, essential, primitive experience which originates beyond the boundaries of the Self. The most sincere and essential 'I' is the metaphysical 'It' and not the 'I'. Paradoxically, the task of the 'I' is to hide the truth from others and especially from the subject's own Self. In this way the subject exerts control over the fact that his or her own mind does not express the truth through thoughts and words. The individual is cut off by the 'It' and continues to live in society with what might be termed a 'shrunken Ego'.

Groddeck considers that the belief in man's great power and will is unfounded, since each person's life is directed by a universal unconscious force, called 'It'. This way, as I have indicated, the 'I' is created by the 'It'. The Ego is actually more passive and less deliberate than one thinks.

The 'It', then, has an important function in imposing a role on the Ego. The Ego 'is a mask used by the "It" to hide itself from the curiosity of mankind' (Groddeck, 1929, p. 41).

According to Groddeck, our effort to think is hampered by the lack of emotional understanding of who we are at the deepest levels of being. When the mind of the individual is cut off from the source of his own emotional experiences, the two parts of the person are split. This can lead to a disintegration of the individual, or to such high levels of excitement or even mania that hinder development, integration and mental creativity.

In describing the process of personalization, Resnik (1999) reconsiders the concept of the 'mask' and specifies the origin of the term 'person'. The Latin word 'person' is derived from the Etruscan '*phersu*', which means 'theatre mask' and, in the Greek language, corresponds to the term '*prosopeion*', meaning 'face containing', transformed into the term 'mask of the person'.

The mask is linked to the person, just as the shadow is linked to the body (Artaud, 1938). The shadow or mask of the body is expressed by the costume that the actor wears. The actor is no longer himself in the play but becomes another person, one that has in effect two bodies, a double set of limbs and an outer semblance which is shown to the audience. According to Artaud, the mask used in theatre is a defensive or deceptive tool; it is a way to reveal some parts of the Self that are normally hidden.

So, just like an actor, the individual shows an image of himself that he has constructed as a character, forged according to the desire to imitate a model of life. In Greek tragedy, the individual may have different masks to use in many representations of himself, but being 'a single person' requires being unique. The duplicity between face and mask, body and clothes, person and character disappears as the overall knowledge of one's Self becomes more complete.

The mask hides the real face with its expressions and can lie and confound others. Primitive populations wore very different masks when fighting with other tribes, in order to confuse or scare their enemies. Certain populations of Papua New Guinea covered themselves with mud (*mudmen*) before battle, so that they would not be recognized as human beings.

Even in our society, in order to avoid the process of personalization, individuals disguise themselves by wearing or possessing clothes or objects that give them a pseudo-personality; for example, they may become followers of a certain fashion designer or a manufacturer of powerful cars.

It is up to the analyst to understand the more specific elements behind the mask by means of the patient's voice and gestures, which escape through the openings of the mask: namely, the eyes and the mouth.

The concept of 'false Self' (Winnicott, 1960) refers in part to the concept of the mask: its function is to mask the child's inner reality. It is a primitive defensive organization, employed when the infant's primary needs are consistently not met. It is the child's revolt against being forced to lead a false existence. It can result in initial physical reactions such as general irritability, digestive disorders, etc. It can also affect how the infant reacts to what arrives from the outside world. The new-born produces a series of artificial relationships that he introjects, pretending they are real and satisfying. The 'false Self' hides the 'true Self'. This organization continues during the rest of his or her life.

In his book *The non-existent knight*, Italo Calvino (1959) describes a medieval knight in a shining, white, immaculate suit of armour. The armour, however, is empty because the knight who owns it, Agigulfo, lives in a constantly defensive position; he only exists through the armour and not as a complex human being. Agigulfo is tough and insensitive, detached from people and things as he protects himself behind his shield. In order to protect his feelings from being fragmented, the armour seems to serve as what might be termed an excitation screen (Ulnik, 2007), though he may occasionally devote himself to looking after others, as a way of masking his own need for attachment. His part in the crusade against infidels was not linked to an ideal; it was a sign of a masked need for attachment.

The analyst has to work hard over long periods of time to find the truth beyond the patient's mask or armour.

4.2 Characteristics of the cases described

The four cases that follow are exemplary of the difficulties in the encounter with such patients, though each case differs in terms of symptoms, behaviour and personal history.

By writing about these cases, I wish to illustrate the various ways in which the suffering of the patients can manifest.

Furthermore, I would like to highlight the importance of the information that emerges from the body when one cannot find connections between psychic meanings and the patient's suffering. This notion allowed me to clarify my initial questions regarding how to overcome the absence of 'real' communication and the feelings of emptiness, driving me to attribute possible meanings only on the signs I could see with my own eyes.

All four cases show the ups and downs of my countertransference experience in dealing with autistic residues and the difficult search for the hidden traumatic experiences responsible for deficits in the Self. In the initial phase of the encounter, there was confusion in the relationship arising from coexisting modes: an 'apparently normal' mode (i.e. customary among people of the same age, gender and social status), and a new, 'neurotic-psychotic like' mode, which brought on strong feelings of disorientation.

My state of mental vacuum gradually gave way to a few points of interest, particular to these cases, driving me to conduct further research. Each case elicited questions and curiosity: for example, the cases of Sara and Irene led my research into the skin as a primitive 'organ of action'.

Other points that sparked my interest were the dominant role of sight and of physical sensations in interpersonal relationships; the lack of connection to thoughts and feelings; the patient's attraction to superficial and apparent aspects of reality and of people; the concept of beauty as the main element in the choice of romantic partners; and the prevalence of action over thought.

Gradually, I was able to understand that the disorienting feeling of 'unrealness' I felt in the encounter with the patients could be explained as their unconscious attempt to transform 'me-person' into an 'inanimate object' which they could shape, position in time and space, and respond to with whatever answers they wished to.

I was finally able to connect my deep emotional discomfort with the patient's transference related to their early experience of unrepresented mental states. Their disorienting experience in the initial encounter with the outside world was being replicated; this was characterized by confusion regarding the limits of the Self, and their lack of faith in a supportive relationship.

These encounters also gave rise to a dual track in the relationship deriving from different levels of integration of parts of the personality: one track was represented by the symptom of a 'desolate emptiness', and the other by the assurances of the defences developed over time.

Finally, all four cases illustrate the need to process countertransference before being able to establish a therapeutic relationship. The alternation between therapeutic interventions and transferal responses has motivated me to reflect on the autistic states and to continue my own self-analysis.

References

Artaud, A. (1938) *Le théâtre et son double*, Paris: Gallimard, 1964 [*The theatre and its double*, New York: Grove Press].
Calvino, I. (1959) *The non-existent knight*, New York: Harcourt.
Groddeck, G. (1929) *The unknown self*, London: C. W. Daniel.
Resnik, S. (1999) *Personne et psychose*, Paris: Editions du Hublot.
Ulnik, J. (2007) *Skin in psychoanalysis*, London: Karnac.
Winnicott, D. W. (1960) 'The theory of the parent-infant relationship', *International Journal of Psychoanalysis*, 41, 585–595.

Chapter 5

Sara
Living on the surface

The title of this chapter, 'Living on the surface', is inspired by an aspect of this patient's personality: Sara focused her interest predominantly on the aesthetic and outward aspects of life and of the world around her. I believe that the difficulty in establishing an emotional relationship with her is linked to primitive experiences of disintegration, and this prompted me to search for the missing part of the Self. The interpersonal relationship remained superficial and was not experienced at a deeper level. By analysing my countertransference, I came to hypothesize a part of a 'non-being Self', buried under an apparently structured superficial Self.

My attempt to transform this superficial interpersonal relationship into a more affective one led me to devote myself to the subject of the skin as a 'bodily organ' and the different levels of symbolization, starting from early sensory experiences. In this work, the hardest obstacles I had to overcome were the patient's toxic mania and her apparent addiction to sensory experiences.

5.1 Sara introduces herself

First phase

This case shows how the life of this patient unfolded over time. Although Sara had previously undertaken some psychotherapy, she seemed to possess absolutely no awareness or knowledge of her childhood un-mentalized experiences. My initial difficulty consisted in recognizing the painful part that was hidden behind the mask Sara had consolidated over the years.

Her previous analyst had sent her to me because of new problems that had arisen with the man she was living with, and a female analyst seemed preferable. As for me, I did not ask for any further information: I usually accept all referrals, reserving the right to decide whether or not to continue with a patient following an initial assessment.

Sara described herself and her social environment in a way that was meant to paint a picture of wealth, social success and competence in various professional and cultural arenas. However, what emerged of her personal life seemed to be more like a list of facts than a real story: a sequence of love affairs that inevitably ended, trips, parties and sumptuous things. In relating these events, I noticed that she lacked any fluctuation of feelings. The number and exceptional nature of all these events seemed to be more important than her internal experience. On the surface, it seemed to be the story of a satisfactory life, rich in human relationships.

When she came for the first time, I observed the way she presented herself. Sara was a thin, middle-aged woman of average height, with the body and face of an adolescent and a questioning and astonished expression. She was wearing a motorcycle helmet and jeans and was well groomed. Her face had regular features, she seemed to 'fit well' in social circles, she was self-assured, quite garrulous and prone to making humorous remarks. She was the third-born after two brothers, and at the time we met she was living with her partner and their son and worked as a freelance journalist.

I immediately saw that her vital interests were related to her attraction towards the superficial aspects of people and things, as well as by her sex addiction.

Initially, the atmosphere was rather unusual. The initial transference seemed cordial though anonymous; subsequently, it seemed to create a climate of refusal and defensiveness. There was no explicit request for help. On the contrary, what prevailed was the desire to disparage and attack me in my role as a professional therapist and as a woman of a different generation. At the same time, Sara would occasionally use language one would use with long-time friends or between adolescents, not considering the difference in roles and positions.

The desire to manipulate the situation emerged in her attempt to establish the rules of the setting, the timings and the fee. She alternated between aggressive attacks and humorous, ironic or seductive remarks. Continuous acting-out persisted for many months. She would arrive very late to the sessions, and she never paid on time.

She gradually revealed her resentment towards her previous analysts, stating that their analysis had been a failure.

She seemed to want to form an alliance with a female therapist in order to share the contempt she was experiencing towards her partner.

During the first meetings the patient tried to scrutinize me to see if I was prepared to meet the challenge and could be trusted. However, apart from the evident symptoms, I also tried to find an emotional contact with the patient. In this case, the request for help was rejected or remained hidden: it was evident that it would take considerable effort to establish a relationship on any other footing than the hypothetical battle to establish a winner and a loser. I felt continually attacked whenever I tried to initiate a relationship, and this prevented me from developing constructive thoughts inside my own mind.

I felt so unable to think that I sensed I couldn't have any reverie regarding Sara or any hypothesis about our work. The term 'reverie' indicates the maternal adaptability in the empathic identification with the infant (Bion, 1962). What was missing here was my holding function. Although I was well aware that the capacity for maternal 'reverie' could only be possible in the absence of anxiety, and that the absence of the state of reverie constituted a traumatic element for the infant, I still felt incompetent and irritated. Despite all my work with psychotic adults and children, through which I became familiar with the patients' omnipotent control of reality, I could only cling to the facts of the moment and await new thoughts, which inevitably failed to come.

Sara, however, appeared as a 'simple' neurotic patient, sufficiently versed in psychological terms and inserted in a normal life.

After the first meetings, the events she related made me wonder if there may have been some partial deficit in her cognitive development that might explain her lack of common sense and strange behaviour.

While I understood her grudges towards analysts in general, it seemed that her way of relating to me, considering her age and socio-cultural level, showed a lack of awareness. I could not understand her inadequate behaviour, which was different from not understanding the content or the ambiguities of what she recounted.

Ogden writes that the analytic relationship is one of the most formal and at the same time most intimate human relationships. Formality is a sign of respect towards the analysand and the analytic process. The intimacy of the analytic relationship is a form of intimacy in the context of formality (Ogden, 1992, p. 175).

I agree with Ogden that, apart from children or adults with psychosis or drug addiction, meeting with an analyst is a situation of intimacy, though it is initially formal. It seemed to me that Sara wasn't able to make a distinction regarding our relationship. Despite the exhibited social normality, Sara's social contact could not be modulated by tact, and this was one of her psychological problems. It was evident that the refusal underlying her behaviour denoted not only a good store of pre-existing hate, but also a sense of profound ambiguity about coming to me for 'help'.

For several months I continued to reflect on my countertransference: it was difficult to contain and understand Sara's fierce aggressiveness and her malignant ironic remarks. It took time because I wanted to take on a way of being in the analysis that could be constructive and genuine. I asked myself how I could maintain the rules of the setting within myself while at the same time tolerating Sara's continuous habit of breaking them. How could I maintain the position of being in charge while she accused me of being a despot? How could I tolerate her attempts to demolish my role and my willingness to help? Was I supposed to endure such an intentionally disturbed atmosphere in my work? Was it a plea for help in order to change something in herself or was it a show of force, challenge? As for me, was my not understanding how to take my usual place in the therapeutic relationship an unbearable narcissistic injury that prevented me from thinking?

In order to manage my negative countertransference, I felt the need to listen without speaking until I reached a serene internal mental state. I considered that time would be an indispensable element in sorting out the situation.

All this brought to mind McDougall's experiences (1989) with so-called 'disaffected' patients. Their request for psychoanalysis is mixed with an attempt to render the emotional experience of the encounter lifeless as well as a denial of their need for help from another person. The continuous disparagement and denigration of the analyst, which implies that there is no hope, paralyzes the analyst and brings feelings of guilt because he or she does not expect the analysis to progress. All this makes the analyst feel frozen and overcome by depressive feelings.

As I tried to tolerate my uncomfortable and painful emotional situation, one day I observed the patient standing in front of me as she was about to enter the door. The position of her head was slightly bent to one side as if posing a question: 'Am I welcome or not?' Although this seemed to clash with her usual behaviour, I felt that the question her body expressed was spontaneous, without the mask. I suddenly associated this expression with my beloved dog who had died several years before. When my dog didn't know what to expect from me – an encouragement or a reprimand – she would remain motionless in front of me, her head bent to one side, ready to move once she grasped the emotions expressed by my face or my voice: a confirmation of affection, an invitation to go for a walk or a talking-to for some mischief.

The black helmet Sara wore when I first saw her, which was part of her mask, had now been replaced by the spontaneity of her body. The association with my beloved dog was illuminating, and put me in contact with my primitive feelings as well as with the patient's real, hidden question: can I be accepted and loved? Which of us was looking for the security of being loved? This association/perception allowed truth of the encounter to emerge, or in other words the reciprocal need of two individuals to communicate without masks.

Second phase

After her suggestion of scheduling the initial meetings on her terms, I proposed to establish a regular day and time for weekly sessions. I suggested continuing the sessions for a few months in order to see whether we could work together. During this initial period, I saw Sara face to face. Although she accepted my suggestion, her habitual tardiness continued for some years!

Ogden (1990, 1992) suggests that when a potential patient phones to enquire about working with the analyst, it is advisable to use the word 'consultation' rather than 'session' so as not to foster the idea of already being in the analytic process.

In establishing the relationship with me, Sara manifested neither her need nor her pain, so I ended up being the only one interested in the analytic work. Sara wondered: 'Why would the therapist be interested in me? Clearly she wants to make money!' Since Sara's previous relationships had been based on control and not on love, she was unable to imagine how two persons could share a truly affectionate alliance.

As Winnicott (1962) stated, it is important – in practising psychoanalysis – to try to remain vital, to be in good condition and to be awake.

I felt lively, wide awake but not in good mental condition. As I waited for the session, I had an uneasy feeling that can best be expressed by the word 'disorientation'. This was due to the difficulty of enduring the fluctuations of the transference that shifted from being playful and seductive to being aggressive and sadistic. It lacked both emotional contact and a constructive mental state. I was unable to feel Sara's pain and motivations since they were hidden well behind her mask of grandiosity or normality. As I listened to Sara's words, I was struck by the enormous effort she was making to elicit a grandiose image meant to spark my envy of her.

I believe that her numerous romantic relationships represented experiences of conquest and success that allowed her to experience the feelings of being welcomed and loved. These relationships, however, did not follow the experience of separation and differentiation from the other and were more likely of a symbiotic nature. Thus they could not be considered fundamental and stable experiences: they dissolved at the thought of an actual choice founded on continuity and commitment, as Sara was not able to imagine long-lasting links of affection.

Indeed, when the thought of continuity, alliance and faithfulness emerged, she broke up with these men. Romantic and sexual relationships were heaven on earth; there were no other preoccupations. She didn't care about the feelings of others, there was no sense of guilt when she rejected someone, never a moment of depression. The other seemed to be used to fill her immediate needs.

When she realized that an affair was set on a collision course, her quickest solution was to show her contempt and totally demolish the other, thus putting the other out of her mind. This was also a continuous warning for me! As a final solution, self-destruction was always better than defeat. Our relationship seemed to rest on a cloud that could move or disappear at any moment. Now and then, she would entertain the idea of ending our relationship, driving me out of her life and thereby making me feel impotent, incompetent, a mere stopgap.

Subsequently, the analytic relationship turned into one of adhesiveness rather than of attachment. Her need was more primitive and, during this phase, my acceptance made it necessary for me to be a reassuring presence. Since I realized there was no idea of an inner space but only of a surface, internalization was going to be difficult. The people around her were so masked by her projections that it was impossible for her to understand the real characteristics of the other, distinct from her own intentions. The inability to feel emotionally secure seemed to have stimulated omnipotence in the rest of the personality.

The production of dreams – though lacking accompanying associations – alongside her need to wait for my interpretations, began to testify to her collaboration and helped me better understand her. At the same time, however, she also wanted to exploit me by taking possession of my thoughts; she continually threatened to end the analysis and did not acknowledge the help I had given her. I became something to use and immediately discard. The separations at the weekends or during my absences were followed by long periods of hostility and acting-out.

From the outset, this work was characterized by her difficulties with interpersonal relationships. What gradually came to mind was the hypothesis of a partial non-existent Self, buried under an 'apparently' or 'falsely' structured Self. Since love and affection were unknown or rejected, the request for communication was only superficial. I become aware of her attempt to transform my person into an autistic object.

She did not perceive her aggressive way of communicating. This did not seem to be a temporary defence mechanism during our sessions; it was rather more an addiction to violence that had slowly developed over the years.

The following months were spent closely observing every fluctuation of the transference and countertransference.

During the first sessions, I felt that Sara's language gave a distorted view of reality: it was full of lies and contradictions that blurred her real thoughts and feelings. While waiting to make sense of the material expressed verbally and continuing to listen attentively to whatever she said, I also took her body language into account.

The body speaks during the session. In the process of personalization that begins from the very first moments of life, the body becomes the receptacle of painful or comforting experiences, and over time it remains a person's means of expression. In the adult, it represents a living memory and constitutes an archaic and essential language (Resnik, 1999). Therefore, observing body language helps us understand the patient, since communication is immediate and sincere.

However, the body is not a symbolic area, and in this case was the hiding place for Sara's primitive pain.

Sara's almost constant symptoms were fatigue and insomnia. In fact, at the start and end of the sessions, she would often yawn loudly to indicate how weary she was of the effort of thinking and how much she desired to regress to a non-thinking state. She would continue to talk even while yawning. Indeed, yawning during a meeting expresses boredom, refusal and disparagement of the presence of the other.

When Sara came into the session, she would forcefully rub her itching eyes at length. The itchiness was justified by an allergic conjunctivitis, dating back to the exact moment Sara learned from medical tests that she was pregnant. Sara had previously suffered from eczema and allergies.

Rubbing her eyes seemed to reveal the shift in her attention from the emerging problems in her mind to the exterior of the body, namely, her skin. Contact with the skin and mucous membranes replaced the acknowledgement of any psychic meaning. Sara failed, or refused, to see the images inside her mind as being connected to the analysis. However, since insight into the internal world requires a process of symbolization, the disorder manifested itself quickly and concretely through the body. In these moments, she could no longer see the studio room, and only experienced bodily sensations. My presence was wiped out and she remained in the darkness.

In dermatology, it is recognized that itching is a symptom equivalent to anxiety at the psychic level, and to pain at the organic level. It is interpreted as being a result of displacement and an extension of anal itching. Freud (1905) used the term 'itching' with reference to sexual excitation.

Considering that the skin is an erogenic zone and scratching an act in search of erogenous satisfaction, itching can be seen as a form of masturbation. (Ackerman, 1938; Pichon-Rivière, 1971) These authors studied the material of patients with eczema from a psychoanalytic point of view, making connections between the patient who covers himself with scabs and the helpless infant that needs maternal protection (see Part I).

In Sara's case, in addition to expressing sensory excitation and obsessive repetition, the severe itching prevented her from paying attention to the psychic problem and shifted the discomfort firmly onto the skin.

I supposed that the problems of the skin and the mucous membranes that emerged during the sessions were meant to express a psychic discomfort that was quite visible yet impossible to communicate through words. These stratagems always occurred when my interventions were felt to be disturbing and thus rejected, but the irritation felt could not be understood and expressed verbally.

Schur (1955) considers itching equivalent to anxiety in general, but particularly ascribes it to feelings of hostility. While at one level itching may be self-punishment, at a deeper level it can be a punishment exerted on an external object, represented here by or on the skin.

Observing cases of patients with dermatological problems undergoing psychoanalysis, Ulnik (2007) shows that aggression towards others is located on the surface of the skin through itching, but this also contains an element of projection connected with exhibitionism; in cases of abuse, the scratching provoked by the itching can be interpreted as the unconscious desire to eliminate the aggressor and make him disappear.

When itching and scratching are used for the purpose of resistance, they represent an obstacle, as Ulnik says, which can be very difficult to eliminate.

During the first years of Sara's therapy, another bodily sign, which was always expressed at the beginning of the sessions, emerged in the way she would make violent, sinister and extremely shrill sounds in order to clear her throat, as well as repeated nasal snorts as if she were trying to expel something. My impression was that she wanted to deliberately and forcefully penetrate my ears. I ascribed the violent way she rubbed her eyes and the intensity of those shrill sounds to both a self-aggressive attack to her body and a cry for help. These guttural sounds were 'sound gestures of the body' lacking any form of symbolization.

Regarding this, Rosenfeld (2006) described an 'expulsive nasal tic' as analogous to the bodily behaviour of drug addicts, who make repeated nasal sounds that he interprets as attempts to expel objects introjected into their bodies.

During the first year of analysis, the predominant topic was sexuality. The one thing Sara said she knew for certain was that sexual desire, stimulated by hormones, was an indication of normality, youth and good health, whereas the absence of intercourse led to desolation and death.

According to Sara, sexual relationships represented the depth of interpersonal relationships, but this depth was intended to be physical, inside the body rather than on the surface. She saw the contact with the skin and mucous membranes, especially with extremely eroticized orifices of the body, as evidence of vital and profound interpersonal relationships.

The need for bodily contact and heterosexual relationships, associated with the consumption of recreational drugs and promiscuity, had become obsessive since her adolescence. These forms of contact, which seemed to exist beyond time and spaces, feelings or mental images, immediately brought Sara into a kind of ecstatic state, detached from real life. Ultimately, they became mixed with deadly sensations.

Tustin (1990) considered drug addiction as the need to be enveloped by sensations of warmth instead of the containment offered by the skin. Without sexual relationships, there would be the emptiness of the 'non-being Self'. It is noteworthy that the orifices represent the point of separation between the skin and the mucous membranes, between the interior and the exterior, indicating differentiation between two persons.

Sara's sex addiction served the purpose of wishing to merge with the other to avoid a terrifying void. But emerging from symbiotic fusion can only in fact be established by developing an object relationship.

Without realizing it, Sara had been imprisoned in an interior tyranny that insisted on the repetition of autistic activities (bodily sensations) to get away from the fear of 'non-being'.

Sara frequently talks about how she shows her affection for others through caresses; these can generally represent feelings of affection, but can also be used for other more deviant intentions, such as in cases of paedophilia! Considering the content and the associations made during our sessions, I can say that the obsessive, repetitive caresses represented not only her need to transmit affection, but also a regressive phantasy of merging with another person, or preventing them from leaving her.

As with all early infant experience, the formation of autistic shapes (Tustin, 1984) originates with softness, which in the baby's mind becomes associated with feelings of security, warmth, comfort and affection. This transformation in the psychic world can only occur when the mother gives affective meanings to the sensory world of the child and to the relationship between them.

During the course of the analysis, some of Sara's psychosomatic disorders, such as insomnia and untreatable gastric pain, became chronic. I gradually came to understand that the body, and in particular the skin, were the depositories of early sensory experiences that had not been transformed into mental states through an object relationship: there was thus a defect in the process of symbolization.

5.2 Spilling and dissolving[1]

Some months passed with weekly meetings, in a situation of uncertainty regarding the continuity of the analytic work. I tried to maintain the idea of continuity within myself, reflecting on the emerging elements. For many sessions, she only talked about the characteristics of other people, her sexual dissatisfaction and her need to have fun. Soon after, she began to suffer from insomnia and anxiety. She called me immediately to book some extra sessions.

Sara's anguish emerged shortly thereafter, confirming my hypothesis of the presence of a primitive, autistic nucleus, accompanied by a state of insufferable catastrophe and loss of identity, Sara told me repeatedly about her suicidal thoughts.

At this point, I re-proposed a regular setting, with three sessions, but she only accepted twice-weekly meetings.

My decision to use the couch in the setting was owing to my need to be isolated and fully concentrated on my feelings: I had to steer clear of excessive projective identification so as to be aware of and acknowledge my own feelings and thoughts. The transition from face-to-face contact to the couch initially provoked in Sara a greater feeling of loneliness, which she had not felt previously. But I think that while Sara 'lost' my face when she moved to the couch, she also took up a new position of being – as it were – in a cradle with the analyst/mother looking down at her. Did she begin to trust in a new internal object because of this more passive and regressive position?

Sara told me she had collapsed into a 'black hole'. She did not know how to save herself. Then the daily anxiety turned into anguish and new bodily symptoms began to appear:

> I feel that I am made of air, I feel like a balloon flying with no string holding me down, I feel like an open tube that connects my mouth to the intestines; I feel like I have a skinless, open hole in my stomach, I'd like to sew it up with some thread; I put my hands on my stomach in order to protect myself and stop my bowels from falling out; I feel like I have a steel vice gripping my liver; I have the terrible sensation of not having an internal space; I feel like a frayed body with no contours.

> My mother didn't have any contact with me, my father used to beat me ... During my sleepless night, I imagine I sew the hole in my stomach, everything is temporary, I can't allow myself to relax, I'm scared that something terrible might happen to my son...

I felt upset thinking about the death of this little boy, but I could not say a word to Sara. I kept my worries to myself, but I did confide in a colleague friend.

Sara felt confused about her whole personality, her lack of identity, fear of disintegration, and all this was accompanied by feelings of catastrophic and persecutory anxiety. She feared she was 'going mad'. Finally, the warrior mask revealed a fragile, sensation-dominated part that had hitherto been hidden.

I became very worried regarding the level of regression and the lack of a centre of gravity. I felt there was no thinking mind inside her body. She described her mood: 'I feel like an astronaut who lost the connection to the spaceship and is in free-fall through the atmosphere. I myself like I was falling into space.'

Bick (1986) described the infant whose projections are not contained by the mother as 'an astronaut in space without a space suit'.

After my previous defensive distance, I now felt the entirety of Sara's despair, and I held the internal image of a protective net that could save her from falling. I felt the urgency of providing emergency care to prevent the danger of dissolution (Reclamation, Alvarez, 1992, p. 53).

After the crisis, many similar dreams appeared in the work with Sara, with situations of danger and fragile maternal support. Recurrent themes included turbulent streams or rivers that sweep onwards; slippery sheets of ice or snow; the sea-bottom filled with drowned children; people without any strength. To outline the development of this first period, I would like to recount two dreams regarding desolation:

1. I am on the bridge over a river with my mother, she tells me to be careful, but at this very moment she falls into the water. I'm upset, I try to run in the direction of the running water, I can touch her, but the current takes her away.
2. My son falls into the water, then emerges again and tries to cling to a rock. I see him and want to plunge into the water, but I am wearing a raincoat and I can't swim. I ask my mother to help me take off my raincoat but my mother doesn't help me. I cry because the little boy doesn't have the strength to survive.

I wonder whether the raincoat might represent a previous waterproof protection against feelings: a wish to be impervious?

Sara also had very different dreams in which she showed extreme courage and possessed the ability to carry out reckless actions to achieve exceptional goals and gain satisfaction through permanent manic excitement. The words she used to describe these dreams were grandiose and hyperbolic.

During the sessions, Sara said she felt less lost, but once she was alone, the feeling of non-existence came back. The sessions continued with an active production of dreams, but always with variable delays, both in arrival time and in payment, accompanied by remarks of mockery and irony.

I felt that these delays represented the permanent devaluation of my work, as if I did not exist. However, I often wondered if underlying the aggression shown in these repeated behaviours was the fact that I had turned into a 'non-existent Self' that could not understand the emotional significance of our interpersonal relationship. At this time, another part of Sara's Self tended to provoke refusals on my part; this was the part that wanted to return to the passive position of the victim, escaping her responsibility in our relationship.

I tried to approach the problem of late arrivals with an explanatory teaching model, emphasizing the loss of valuable time we needed to analyse her problems. I also tried to express my own regret about this wasted time. I told her about my anxiety when I waited for her. In response, Sara said that, when someone was late for a business meeting, she was happy because she could quietly read the newspaper. My regret appeared to her to be false or incomprehensible.

At this point, I decided to wait before interpreting the acting-out and to concentrate on the dream material. I believe that, even in therapeutic work with psychotic patients or those with a severe deficiency of the Self, we have to work with what we have in order to reach the patient, rather than stick rigidly to the theoretical models of interpretation of analytic schools (Cremerius J., personal communication in supervision, 1980).

In retrospect, we might consider that this outbreak of acute symptoms affecting both body and mind occurred when the patient was able to finally find the security of a cosy nest, where she could deposit her suffering and be understood.

Numerous dreams followed. There were what she called the 'butcher shop' dreams, filled with rubbish, faeces, dead bodies, dismembered and unexplainably abandoned corpses, or fierce fights between animals. She related other dreams in which she killed people, cutting their heads off with a sword in anger and with no sense of guilt. No associations emerged: these dreams appeared to me to be primitive fantasies, full of violence, and there was no thought that they might be significant and we could think about their meaning. Human bodies were not sexually differentiated; they were merely pieces of bodies that belonged to no one.

Only later I thought that this desire to kill in the dreams was connected to a narcissistic structure in which killing represented an excitement that replaced the possibility of having a psychic life. The desire to kill, which was also the desire to kill her 'Self', was the only element that apparently gave her energy (Symington, 2007).

It was only later, through different dreams, that she started to become aware of her past violent actions.

Sara's perception of her body during the crisis appeared to be disintegrating and required continuous control on her part, for fear that she would disappear completely.

Autistic experiences in language, body image and dreams

In the adult patient, the outbreak of a crisis related to the loss of identity and the sensation of a dissolving body confirms the hypothesis of this particular aspect of the autistic experience, as documented in work with autistic children. Moreover, the evidence given by adults through language provides greater elements of knowledge than those provided by autistic children.

Sara refers to feelings of loss of contact with surrounding reality and with her body, underlining her difficulty in expressing these feelings. They are unknown sensations, or sensations that have never been recognized and are therefore difficult to convey to others with commonly accepted language.

The word 'death' was usually not employed in the literal sense of the word, but indicated a dark environment devoid human beings: a 'sense of death'. At the same time, language describing actual death was not connected with sad feelings, but rather represented a return to a situation of inertia.

The crisis of bodily dissolution reproduces the experience of early undifferentiated states in which unthinkable anxieties lead to a feeling of having lost parts of one's body. In the absence of sufficient support, and with the inability to control the outside world, the baby experiences a state of terror that becomes magnified and ends in catastrophe. The 'black hole' represents the first depressive experience (Tustin, 1972, 1981) and the inability to acknowledge bodily separation. Tustin (1981, p. 11) described the 'black hole' as a subjective experience of space: it represents for the infant the terror of disconnection with the mother who had previously been felt to be a part of his body.

Grotstein (1990, p. 257) points out that the experience of the black hole is an 'experience of the awesome force of powerlessness, of defect, of nothingness, of a state of "zero-ness" expressed not just as static emptiness, but as an implosive, centripetal pull into the void'. That space is felt as the presence of an inhuman and malevolent absence that must be eliminated from awareness.

The first bodily sensations are fundamental in establishing one's identity and one's survival. The repetition of sensations and their satisfaction triggers the learning of idiosyncratic shapes (Tustin, 1972). A cluster of sensations beginning with the combined nipple–tongue experience gives the impression of merging with the mother, and it is impossible to differentiate one from the other.

The configuration of these bodily experiences as forms of contact denotes a state of safety represented by autistic shapes. Subsequently, the attachment to other sensory couplings in the bodily image, such as faeces–intestines and penis–vagina, will take on the same notion of being merged and undifferentiated. Symptoms such as persistent constipation and sex addiction can be seen in this context.

When the absence of continuity in the experience of early sensory couplings occurs at a very early period or in a traumatic way, the result is a feeling of the body breaking into pieces. This is followed by the sensation of falling into a vacuum at the centre of an external, unknown world. The experience is that of being left to fall into an empty space with nothing to hold on to.

The outbreak of such crises in an adult demonstrates the representation of such buried experiences that occur during important emotional events, such as marriage, divorce, pregnancy or mourning. These experiences cannot be mentalized, owing to the immature psychic state of the early infantile period or to the inability to symbolize. The dreams of these patients relate to fantasies of a non-mentalized world filled with primitive sensations.

Sara's emotional crisis of depersonalization, which occurred after having agreed to enter into analysis, highlights a disorder of her body image and the absence of containment by a skin that could enclose her. Since her identity lies in the concrete form of the body, the sense of non-existence is accompanied by the fear of bodily disintegration. The idea of losing her identity is concretely embodied in feeling frayed, with blurred boundaries.

Anxiety is then a psychic phenomenon that is concretely transformed into a hole in the stomach. In the analytic sessions, it is Sara's hand, rather than her mind, that tries to contain her intestines and keep them from falling out. The idea of being a tube going from the mouth to the intestines demonstrates the primitive experience of being unable to keep any external element 'outside', nor distinguish between one bodily organ and another.

Concerning the body, one particular dream refers to an abnormality in the body of a young girl.

> I am with a mother whose child is playing with my son. I notice that the upper part of the child's body is missing, leaving only the lower part and her legs, which keep on skipping. I'd seen a children's cartoon similar to this image. I ask the mother to explain this strange situation and she tells me that even during her pregnancy she knew that her daughter would be born this way, but since she wanted a baby girl at all costs she decided to give birth to the baby. Although I was astonished by this pathological relationship between mother and daughter, watching those tiny legs nevertheless touched me.

I want to point out that here we have a child with no head nor heart, only legs, intestines and genitals. Even the arms that express what the mind decides to do are missing. However, just as for the patient/mother of the dream, it was essential to give birth to this child. But the mother of the dream had accomplished the violence of her will in giving life to a headless body. The patient associates this with how skilfully she herself can work with her hands, and how proud this makes her feel. Sara does not understand my hint regarding the absence of the head and heart. At that time, highlighting the absence of the mind seemed to be premature. I feared it might be experienced as too bewildering.

In a subsequent dream, there seemed to be a problem regarding the joints of one part of the body and the loss of a function.

> I'm with a friend at the seaside where children are playing. When I return to the beach, I notice that I've got a wound on the upper part of my leg near the femur. I'm like those plastic dolls with detachable legs. I'm worried: as a temporary measure, I tie a scarf around my leg. I want to bring my motorcycle down some steps but I realize that I'm not able to do it any more.

I took this to be an attempt to reproduce an image of a mechanical body and the doubt about being able to maintain a male identification.

Recurring themes in the dreams

Falling into a vacuum

> I fall abruptly from an aeroplane along with my father, mother, and brothers. The prospect of imminent death does not cause me any pain, but I feel sad because I am alone while the other four are holding hands.

Here she talks about her feelings of being abandoned, although in reality she had been well looked after.

Lack of support

> I'm walking in the snow with my family. We're on the bridge of a mountain and by dint of walking in dangerous areas I slide down and end up in an escarpment. Then I fall into the ice-cold water. I freeze and then have to change my clothes.

Indescribable terrors

Sara's internal world was populated by monster-individuals. The belief in unknown worlds, supernatural and unpredictable forces and people filled her imagination and dreams.

Many dreams were full of terror, with supernatural entities that obstructed her movements. These creatures streaked through space without being recognized or captured. Many dreams represented weak individuals or children being tortured or brutally killed. She called them 'bloodthirsty and apocalyptic dreams'.

The unknown part of the unconscious, full of terrifying elements, emerged during Sara's sleep.

> ... I'm with my son on the snow, he slides over but I grab him and save him; but then I feel that some arms are trying to grasp my legs, maybe it was a zombie, something supernatural and diabolical anyway, but I manage to get free and save myself.

> ... I'm with some people and their faces suddenly turn into the faces of devils with sharp teeth. I'm paralyzed with terror. Then I'm at the home of a friend who is a psychoanalyst. She has a toiletry bag with many cosmetics and brushes that she uses with water ('Why only with water', I wonder to myself?). Although she is much older than me, her skin is beautiful. I think I too should have all these things in my toiletry bag.

> ... there's a man that has kept a corpse in a closed room for six years. You (the analyst) are a part of the scientific police force, and you explain that keeping a corpse in the house might be harmful to one's health since it produces toxins.

Here we have the appearance of an anonymous corpse and I hypothesize that the dehumanized aspects of the dream represent the absence of individuality and gender differentiation.

> I'm in a hotel in a city with a port, but I'm not on a ship. I'm worried about certain invisible presences. I sit on the bed and put my feet on the floor. I feel a sticky substance holding me back, and there is something pulling me under the bed. The person in charge stays with me to help me and is trying to find the meaning of what is happening, and then finally says that the police should be called. Nobody understands what's happening.

Here we can see the beginning of a helpful relationship with me:

> I'm in a terrifying landscape in front of a deep lake. The lake is sad with no people in or around it. It could be the lake of death, and thinking about it makes me shudder. It was as if it was something hanging between two worlds. I was with 'X', a psychiatrist friend of mine, a strange fellow. This dream is set in Africa. We're in an inlet between two rocks; perhaps we're having a snack. In the distance we see a tyrannosaurus approaching; it's one of those very scary dinosaurs with a big white head. It's at least two metres tall. When it gets near us, I'm scared to death, but my friend – who'd been eating his snack, strokes it and gives it some friendly pats on the snout, just as if it were a dog, so that it would get out of the way.
> I think my friend is very brave. Suddenly in the darkness the water lightens, a ball-shaped fish comes up to the surface with a light. I become completely petrified, the dark night is coming, and we run away.

Violence

Many of these dreams had violent content with no clear motivation, unaccompanied by any feelings. There were many dreams filled with unidentified corpses, with undifferentiated genders, and these almost photographic scenes of killings occurred frequently.

> I'm with a group of people and we don't know where to sleep. I remember a hotel that I used to know well, and we go there. I see now that there's a kind of cage – no, a kind of space filled with some nice, small, chubby dinosaurs that arouse my tenderness. They're the offspring of the huge dinosaurs. Suddenly, a cook holding a sword pierces one of these baby dinosaurs and takes it to the kitchen to skin and cook.

There would be associations to these dreams, after a long silence.

> After a trip to China, I remember enormous frogs that were killed in the market that continued to jump even after their heads had been cut off.

Terrible. I was shocked by seeing turtles without their shells, just in their flabby skins.

I think that the skin of the small dinosaurs, which was torn up so violently, as well as the immature skin of the shell-less turtles represented a weak, skinless and helpless state.

These dreams hold signs of abuses committed towards the young offspring of animals or children who cannot defend themselves and are at the mercy of violent adults. Sara, too, is aware of her own aggression.

The fascination of surface and the role of skin

I was soon struck by the prevalence of Sara's interest in the superficial aspects of people and things, which had determined every choice in her life up to that point. Even the 'material' of dreams was made up of images she especially appreciated for their surface features: the descriptions of the visible quality of things were meticulous.

In Italian, the word 'beautiful' ('bello') is almost always used alongside the word 'carino'. This word is derived from the Italian 'caro', or 'dear', which contains an emotional element. We use this diminutive to indicate the world of childhood. We can think of a primitive analogy or confusion between beautiful and dear.

There are many adjectives which are used to describe various situations. For example: shiny and bright objects, delightful decorations, opaque water of a lake – be it motionless or dark, an unusually beautiful fish full of luminosity in the dark, etc. For Sara, these superficial visual elements represented interesting and attractive features that held no particular affective meaning.

The pleasure given by the sight of and physical contact with these surfaces she considered to be 'beautiful' was connected to fetishism and to an obsessive mental organization with patterns of order and perfection. Moreover, she adhered to certain conventional social standards, making use of repetitive and reassuring elements that she shared with other people. For example, the individual pieces of household furniture, chosen according to her aesthetic tastes, evoked in Sara an image of well-being and happiness in the family despite the absence of an affective atmosphere.

Here we can see the importance of the concept of the mask in relation to other people and the environment (see Chapter 4, Section 4.1: The mask of the Ego).

The surface of people and objects (skin, somatic forms, clothing) became of utmost importance in establishing so-called romantic or friendly relationships: the choice of partners was based on 'aesthetic form', meaning their physical appearance; just as the break-ups, once final, were attributed to physical defects or imperfections, or to the ex's untidy homes.

This superficial view of the world coincided with the more general social environment around her, and she felt reassured in mirroring herself in their exterior standards.

I should point out that Sara's tendency to observe and appreciate the beauty and the superficial aspects of the external world, without differentiating between persons or objects, had nothing to do with the aesthetic experience, which produces transformative emotions and associations through the contemplation of works of art. Sara's attitude seemed to express merely a concrete world of surfaces without any depth. Her language seemed to refer to this concrete world of surfaces and lacked what might be termed 'emotional depth'.

Regarding one of Sara's break-ups, Liberman's concept (Liberman et al., 1982) helped me understand her predicament. In fact, the separation from her partners was not a painful loss of the other as a thinking and affectionate person; indeed, her experience was like tearing away part of the surface of her body from the other's. It was painful to break away from the exterior of the admired companion, or from his physical presence, even though living with him had been extremely problematic. According to Liberman's conceptualization, Sara suffered the loss of the 'beautiful' aspects of him and his refined objects, rather than the loss of a relationship with a thinking, loving and suffering person. In the face of a separation, Sara defended herself by devaluating the other person in the couple (the person who was leaving), a defence designed to avoid falling into depressive feelings. Suffering a loss meant mainly the absence of a continuous presence, of aesthetic satisfaction and of control over the other.

Sara's stories transported me into a world of beautiful objects, luxury and fashion, meant to arouse my envy and to show her own superiority. She never reported any fluctuations of feelings in her life, never any experiences of pain or loss.

While the skin normally provides containment and energy, Sara often complained of being cold and feeling tired and without energy, as if her skin did not perform its protective function.

Both in dreams and in reality, Sara often described malformations of the skin due to abnormal over-production. Since these kinds of congenital malformations originate from defects in the development of the foetus, the focus on these abnormal images evokes primitive sensorial malfunctions. The discovery of these abnormal pieces of bodies evoked feelings of disgust and death: they included random fingers, ears in abnormal locations and surplus nipples.

Dreams about skin

> ... Then I go to the bathroom, I take my time because I'm removing the blackheads from my skin. While squeezing them out, a small animal emerges, similar to an iguana or a small dinosaur, and I throw it away.

My reflections on this content are based on all the previous associations and developments of the session. The blackheads spoil the perfection of the skin and have to be eliminated, but are transformed into prehistoric animals as a trace of a primordial era that Sara does not want to consider.

The skin still retains this evidence of primitive experience.

> ... We then go and find a lot of people in my apartment lying on the bed, along with a dermatologist who does not notice my small razor wounds, but makes his own diagnosis. I ask him to whisper, so that the others do not hear.

The skin presents wounds that are difficult to identify, produced by a sharp, aggressive tool. Perhaps the wounds are the results of painful experiences unacknowledged in her previous therapeutic contacts.

> ... The skin is the site of stroking, I have an atavistic thirst for caresses, without them I'm like a fish out of water that dries up and has to be put back into the water again.

> ... Now I understand that I am at a stage in life where I'm changing my skin, I never imagined this would happen ...

The psychic transformations are still located in the skin rather than in the mind.

> ... I go to the spa with X and at the entrance, there's a very demanding receptionist who makes us fill in forms with our personal information, but the information is wrong and we have to redo the forms. I think: what a bureaucratic idiot. I'm so angry I'm about to explode, but I restrain myself. I put on a protective cream, the same one that X puts on before going into the pool in order to prevent the chlorine from worsening his dermatitis ... For me, the spa represents regression, I just love going into the warm water. I need to relax, my body is hypersensitive. If I have a bad feeling, I feel it in my body.

The spa represents analysis, where the organization (the idiot analyst) imposes rules and she complains about the fact that she has to repeat elements of her past. The analysis is not just a hot, relaxing bath; one has to withstand the chlorine, which protects against infections but is also an irritant. This dream takes place at the beginning of the four weekly sessions. With such frequent contact, one must protect oneself, and there may be new and irritating points of view that are difficult to accept.

The sensory meaning of the skin and the mucous membranes replaces the mental world

As has already been noted in the previous paragraphs, since Sara's adolescence, her demand for physical contact and heterosexual relationships, associated with drug consumption, became an almost obsessive need. Skin contact, especially through the body orifices, which were extremely erotized, was of utmost importance, and confirmed to her the presence of profound interpersonal relationships.

There were no fantasies, projects or long-lasting emotional bonds between Sara and her sexual partners. This went on, it seemed, interminably. Sara's deathly feelings emerged; it seemed as if the real world no longer existed. Without realizing it, Sara was obliged to repeat these autistic activities in order to escape from the feeling of 'non-being'.

This early pseudo-genitality can be seen as a defence against the experience of an internal emptiness and as a way of regulating interpersonal distance. It can also be regarded as a substitute attachment to the penis instead of to the breast.

The drug addiction represents the need to be enveloped by sensations of warmth, which replace the usual kind of containment by the skin (Tustin, 1990).

I think that, in Sara's case, these repeated caresses served to soothe the painful wounds of early non-emotional contact.

Towards mentalization

Over time, Sara slowly started to observe the scheduled sessions and payments, and followed the rules we had agreed on. A great production of dreams followed, though these produced associations that for the most part showed no clear evidence of meaning. Although my comments were rarely taken into account, I continued to have a wide range of associations regarding Sara's dreams and I offered her my thoughts.

Despite the fact that during the session Sara would describe a general sense of both physical and mental well-being, when she left the session it was as if no representation of the experience remained in her mind.

During the first period of the work, expressions of anger and violence against others prevailed, and her way of speaking was evacuative. Her language was immediate and she didn't think things through. In the transference, irritation or contempt was expressed through ideological reasoning against psychoanalysis, through late payments and by never arriving on time. She also gave me detailed descriptions of her visits to alternative doctors, oriental healers, shamans. She followed their remedies without being concerned about upsetting me, even though it also seemed to be a means of challenging me. She thought that the shaman's advice was faster and more accurate than my interpretations. The attacks and devaluations of the analyst often moved far away, as if they were unconnected with our work in any real way. Although we know that acting-out conveys the inability to express aggressive feelings directly, it was nevertheless meaningful. I therefore patiently waited and observed.

As the analysis progressed, the transference changed from a fight to a sort of union, as if we were a single person, with a similar way of feeling and judging. She asked me for my opinion or to confirm her ideas, using a confidential tone: her sentences ended with the question 'isn't that so?'. The differences between us emerged only when the problem of the payment for missed sessions reminded her that there was indeed a difference between us.

Her most frequent communication described her intense sensory impressions and bodily states, rather than her thoughts. Sara's recurring topic was that of her sexual life, determined by hormonal changes, which she considered to be the only factors responsible for people's happiness and behaviour.

The deprivation that she experienced as a child became an obsession to which she returned many times. Given the rigidity of her thoughts, however, no internal transformation appeared possible.

Sara considered analytic work to be iatrogenic in the sense of making her sick and causing a depressive state. In this way, the analysis was, she thought, wilfully persecutory. She felt that my interpretations deprived her of any sensory satisfaction. They described a sad life in a way she felt to be both critical and dogmatic.

Thinking of experience of motherhood led to the re-emergence of her own primitive maternal bond. The symptoms of dissolution of the body and the Self overlaid the previous manic and narcissistic organization. She now seemed mentally confused, in a psychotic mental state.

The 'absence' she had felt in many sexual encounters revealed her previous internal state of mind, based merely on close bodily and sensory contacts in the absence of a successfully internalized object. The primitive fantasies of fusion and the terror of having a separate identity prevailed and emerged in the form of the problems Sara experienced regarding sexual identification.

Communication with the analyst was possible only by sharing the same kind of ideas or feelings. In my countertransference, I felt close to her regarding the interpersonal experience, and I communicated this to her; at the same time, however, I also offered a different point of view. In this way, I created a differentiation between us, namely, sharing ideas and overlapping, as well as partly differentiating her from myself.

Four sessions a week

The request to increase the number of sessions to four accelerated the analytic work. Perhaps, however, this change was more a desire for adhesive proximity with me than a wish to exchange thoughts. It was very difficult to speak about the transference. It seemed that we were both inside the same membrane without any differentiation. If I had not allowed her to have this experience – namely, the kind of closeness she imagined as the only way to stay together – Sara would have ended the relationship. Interrupting any relationship that might threaten her autonomy and certitude was her way of managing disagreement: she would tell me and everyone else to go to hell and just leave!

What loomed in sight were two risks: the first was the internal danger of dissolution, and the second was the exterior danger of being rejected. The object relationship existed only in the presence of the other, while in absence it completely disappeared. Due to the difficulty of keeping the absent object in mind, she could not construct an internal representation of a stable relationship over time.

Through the material, I pointed out that her behaviour was a response to strong primitive emotional needs, and suggested that other factors were necessary in adult relationships, such as tolerance, patience and understanding of feelings of others. In her past, she could not accept, or did not know, the word 'patience'. When she faced obstacles, she could only distance herself from the other by running away. Due to her projective identification, she feared that my patience and tolerance towards her would also end. If she rejected me, then of course – she reasoned – I would ultimately reject her.

Falling into the 'black hole' (the term she herself used when she slipped into desolation) represented the greatest fear when she was away from me. She lost both hope in the future and any faith in her own psychic strength. She had many dreams in which she had no power to save herself from falling into water, or she had nothing to hold on to. She expressed frequent fantasies and dreams of death and mummification; a deathly atmosphere pervaded these frightful scenarios. Initially, the background of these dreams was represented by cold icy deserts that subsequently became torrid sand dunes where human presence was rare. Aspects of strength were represented only in scenes of aggression and violence. Feelings regarding human relationships could be intense, but these adhesive attachments could then be completely erased without any feelings of guilt.

Painful situations in dreams were expressed as an experience of 'non-being'. There was no idea of continuity over time nor distance in space: the object disappeared when not in view, namely, it was absent. She recognized that she could in fact think about the continuity of our meetings, but at times she said she could 'no longer find the energy or strength' to come to the sessions. She felt that her energy was something concrete in her body with no emotional component.

When I went away on holiday, she experienced my physical distance as a form of abandonment, thus re-living past experiences of absence. Sara felt extremely angry about having to undergo the separation. But wishing to be close to another person meant acknowledging her dependence on them. In the past, it was she who had abandoned the other, without bothering about their feelings.

Initially, she was terrified that thinking about meanings in analysis and remembering her past life would only lead to desolation and destruction. However, we can see the gradual changes in the analysis and in our relationship in the dreams that follow. '... In the depths of the sea, beyond a particular area populated by magnificent tropical fish, there is darkness with only stones, sand and no animal life.' As the analysis proceeded, she became frightened by the idea of being nullified, and feared the deflation of narcissism; this was linked to a world of death.

> ... are you familiar with Jules Verne's Journey to the Centre of the Earth? It's painful to arrive at the secret room that had never been imagined. Despite the heaviness, I'm happy to have found the room, but I'm afraid the pain could lead to cancer so I go and have blood tests taken. It seems to me almost a profanation to say so ... great white sharks are blind ... Now I feel better, I feel more solid and often have physical ailments that usually clear up ... I'm always afraid of the inevitable. I'm not afraid of death, in fact, I think it would be a release from difficulties...

I try not to leave her alone in this desolation, where the analysis is felt to be painfully digging into her in a judgemental way. I say that the archaeologist/analyst digs to find life and the treasures of the past, and even if they are sometimes broken fragments, they can explain important events. Although they do not always find something that is clear, their interest is focused on enhancing the value of what remains. In other cases, in deserts or barren lands, the aim of digging is to find precious water. By digging into the past we find personal experiences that bear witness to different periods and levels of personality. For example, in the first days of life, when the mind is still undeveloped, we discover traces of our early bodily experiences.

Sara's view that our relationship only led to useless and possibly harmful explorations meant that she was unable to move away from disappointing primitive experiences, and she had to deny any hope for the future. Moreover, it was also a way to disparage me and transform me into an enemy.

I suggested that the blindness of white sharks was also hers; but now, through the analysis, she recognized her blindness and had to move the spotlight from the behaviour of other people to her own inner world. This new vision was what was making her sight blurry.

> ... a new profound part of me sustains me and another makes me doubtful. I'm afraid that digging deeper would make me see the pain, I'm afraid of being overwhelmed. I removed some pieces of myself in order to grow up, I would have been annihilated before ... the danger is the unknown feelings in my mind, that are like unknown supernatural and esoteric phenomena.

Another dream that attests to the awareness of her inner world is the following: 'There are two bulls in a barbed-wire pen, wounding each other with their horns, pushing each other against the fence, and eventually dying from their wounds. I am shocked by the foolishness of this violence.' The associations of this scene caused her much pain, thinking about the foolishness of aggression for its own sake. The previous omnipotence which had been her defence in childhood began to diminish through the analytic work. Now she felt pain at seeing the stupidity of some of the actions she had taken with no connection between thoughts and feelings.

The following dream accurately describes further development in the acknowledgement of her behaviour.

> ... After being assaulted by a motorcyclist on the road, I angrily throw his screwdriver into the sea in revenge. He wants me to give it back to him so I go into the water and look for it among the algae deep down in the water; they are not slimy. I find objects such as knives and scissors, a beautiful pair of stainless steel scissors, one dating back to the seventeenth century, a small, precious box with a compass embedded on the lid and inside a map, perhaps of Africa. I think it probably belonged to a drowned explorer who had been attacked by pirates. I find wonderful things...

The human relationship within the analysis is almost incomprehensible to her, because it goes beyond the concrete physical laws that regulate objects. In a subsequent dream she is amazed by my 'superhuman ability' to juggle her incomprehensible and unrepeatable thoughts.

> You were juggling small geometric crystals and the degree of skill and dexterity in this game was such that it made me think of your supernatural powers that went beyond the laws of physics and, in particular, the classic schemes of psychoanalysis. I wonder why I am so tied to you that I give up going on holiday.

Describing therapies with chronically depressed or desperate children, Alvarez (1992) talks of idealization being a necessary phase, and indeed it is a major step in this patient's development. Obviously, we have to differentiate this kind of idealization from a manic defence: at that very moment, I was experiencing a genuine emotional contact.

The massive projective identifications of the past had made her feel certain that she could actually understand the feelings of other people. But in the end, she couldn't even recognize her own feelings. Although her need to be accepted was fundamental, she was always waiting passively for others to give meaning to her life, without being able to know what she herself needed.

This problem persisted in the relationship with me. The problem that arose was: how can we keep the right distance when the patient is hypersensitive to rejection while also maintaining independence and separateness? How can I interpret her aggression in the transference without pushing her away and thus endangering our fragile relationship?

We must therefore distinguish between addiction and adhesiveness with regards to the analyst from a real communicative relationship. The relationship may appear to be intense, aiming to enslave the analyst and make her powerless. Sometimes the patient uses seductive and controlling stratagems by saying things like, 'You're the best analyst in the world!'

> I had a dream, I don't know if it is good or bad. I dreamt of you. I was in a kind of hospital, usually I dream of the same kind of places. I was pregnant and I gave birth to a very small baby, like this (she holds up her hand), it could have been a doll; I didn't give the baby the importance of a baby. While wandering in this hospital, I found you and I immediately remembered that I had forgotten the baby somewhere. I run to the car and I find the baby there, but I am afraid that the baby is dead. You want to take the baby in your hands and try some skilful manoeuvres and massages to reanimate him, but you can't bring him back to life. You only manage to make him as large as a normal baby.
>
> Then the setting of the dream changes: I am in Berlin, in my ex fiancé's house, with him and my friend. I teach them how to clean the house and the old paintings on the wall with a strong jet of streaming water, like a virtual stick. I don't know where the dust goes. When I broke up with this man, I didn't want to leave anything in his house, but in the dream I don't worry about not removing everything, and I leave some dishes there. I don't care any more.

Sara offered these associations:

> I feel that something in me has been born from our relationship, because I can remember you as a real person even when I am not here with you. Before I thought of you only when I was desperate. The baby was too small to be forgotten and left alone, but I remembered him as soon as I saw you. In the dream, I thought that I usually don't feel guilty when I don't look after something. I think now of my past violence, it was only a way of getting rid of obstacles that got in my way. No one urged me to reflect on my actions. I couldn't even speak to my mother; when I was 17 I didn't think about anything. I had an analyst when I was 30, but he didn't help me, I've always been too superficial.
>
> When I was with my ex fiancé in Berlin, I dreamed that I had a little girl with short, deformed and flabby legs: in fact I left my fiancé because he was the one who had short legs.

Some dreams showed gradual modifications in the transference.

> I feel a strange sense of gratitude towards you, because I can tell you everything about me. I tell you things I've never told anyone. When I was a little girl I didn't think of myself, I often thought that people could disappear or die. Here with you I feel a welcoming, soothing thought.
>
> … I'm afraid of wrongly interpreting facts: I always mistook love for weakness, I regarded men who were affectionate as too clingy. I mistook affection for a crushing weight on me.

At times and with great difficulty, I did manage to use all my sweetness, but it was so infuriating! I can't accept it all. I don't identify with a fawning female who depends on a man. I can't even imagine it: that total dedication makes me sick to my stomach. Such behaviour would only be appropriate towards one's children.

As the analytic work progressed, it became possible to address the issue of mistaken gender identification that had influenced her choices when she was young, as well as her relationships with men.

Considering her primitive experiences of emotional solitude, lack of protection and the terror represented in the image of the black hole, we can suppose that gender identification was problematic and confused.

When Sara became aware of her narcissism, there was an enormous change in her personality. The picture that emerged from this new assessment of her past consequently led to a depressive phase.

In order for her to have a sense of her identity, it is conceivable that Sara obsessively collected relationships that aroused physical sensations in order to experience a sense of vitality and feel that she possessed a separate 'oneness'. There was no idea of an interior space, but only the surface, which was impossible to internalize.

This might be the reason behind the failure of previous analytic attempts.

As the interpretative work progressed, it brought about an enrichment of thought, with Sara's awareness of the need to make an internal change. It became clearer that she needed to break down past defences. The enormous narcissistic construction of her personality had posed many difficulties: it was hard for her to consider herself in a critical light.

Several years into the analytic work, she dreams:

I am in my city and I sense a different smell in the air that reminds me of a childish sensation felt in the mountains. I think that it is different from the usual smell and that the air has improved, given the perennial high pollution levels in the city. The scene changes, and I'm in my house where I'm rearranging my things and I'm undecided whether to throw away all the half-used sun-creams, because I think they are too old. I find one that's almost new, and I'm sorry to throw that one away. Then I find plastic pieces of various shapes, some could be containers, some are sharp and I throw them all down the toilet, because I don't need them any more. I am amazed that they can be pushed down by the force of the water.

The defences adopted against spending too much time in the hot sunshine and getting sunburnt again refers to the surface of the body. Doubts arise regarding keeping sun lotions (the mask) or sharp objects (aggressiveness) as protective defences – and how much do they really protect anyway? The useless plastic pieces refer to artificial and worthless substances.

It took many years to finally combine the feelings and thoughts in Sara's mind in a constructive and personal way. The initial analytic relationship turned into an exciting, moving and touching experience, once it became sincere and filled with feelings.

Fluctuations in countertransference during analysis

When I think about Sara, I remind myself once again that these patients have a 'normal' or neurotic-like area of social behaviour alongside behaviours which emerge as the analytic relationship is being established, which implicate a deficiency of Self.

I would like to divide the characteristics of Sara's patterns of behaviour into three successive periods.

The first period was particularly difficult since I was, as it were, under the 'anaesthetic effect' that the patient projected into me. She brought a confused message to her analysis: she had the perception of profound suffering but was unable to confess it to either herself or to others. My difficulty was in sensing that the language she used led to distortions of reality, lies and evasiveness, which blurred her real state of mind.

The repeated acting-out put me in the condition of not really being in contact with the patient in the session and colluded with my own feelings of impotence. For example, although she always arrived late and paid late, none of my explanatory hypotheses were taken into consideration and were therefore useless. I understood that in order to come out of the prison of this impotent state of mind, I just had to contain and 'live with' the inconvenience of her tardiness, accepting the fact that she was unable to stop this behaviour since she lacked a thinking mind. At the same time, as I have previously said, I had to maintain within myself the rules of the setting.

The development of the therapeutic situation depends on the possibility of having a point of contact between the feelings of both participants. For a long time, the emotional encounter consisted only in sadistic attacks masked with humour, and they triggered my own defensive narcissistic countertransference. Her requests were about changing the rules of our meetings and reducing my fees, but they were also attempts to intrude into my life. My countertransference led me to question my self-confidence as a therapist.

In discussing sadistic behaviour seen in the treatment of children with psychotic traits, Alvarez (2012) describes the need to pay close attention and monitor every moment of the session in order to overcome a clash with this type of pathology. These patients compete with the analyst, not on the level of thoughts and affection, but on the level of bravado, strength and the ability to not be taken in. This type of work requires time and close attention.

One might start to wonder: 'What is the patient doing to me?'

The countertransference – namely, the set of the analyst's unconscious feelings prompted by the patient – was fully discussed by Bion (1955, 1961). He points out that it is the task of the analyst to analyse these feelings within himself/herself and not use them directly in the consulting room. This requires having to go over one's own feelings and make sense of them, for example, by keeping in touch with one's own hatred instead of expressing it, thinking of it as being inside the analyst's mind instead of shaking it off like a ping pong ball towards the patient (Symington, 2007). Keeping the feelings of both patient and analyst inside allows the analyst to work through the information provided by the patient, whereas the expulsion of these feelings might cause harm to both. Only the containment of these mental states makes it possible to come up with fruitful interpretations. This, of course, links again to Bion and the idea of the communicative nature of projective identification.

So the analyst has to be careful not to immediately put himself in a position of making negative or moral judgements (Symington, 2002, 2007).

The analyst's empathy and insight emerge by identifying with the child-like aspects of the patient's Self. This should bring about an interaction that makes it possible to work in an analytic way. In the case of emotionally blocked patients, this is difficult. However, one must take into consideration that the patient mobilizes in the analyst areas of his own primitive infantile experiences, where psychotic anxieties reappear. Not acknowledging the awakening of these personal areas of primitive experience can trigger the impression of being 'antitherapeutic' and this then makes it impossible to understand the needs of the patient. Consequently, what occurs is a vicious cycle of thoughts that are immobilized.

Concerning the analyst as an empty container open to the patient's questions, Bion (1967) invites us to 'think through images' rather than to use theoretical concepts.

I was able to enter into a relationship with Sara only through containment, my patience and willingness to wait, and the sudden insights that emerged in watching the position of Sara's body or expression.

This association between the position of Sara's head and that of my dog (see Section 5.1, 'First phase') appeared in my mind as a sudden enlightening moment, considering that my dog had died some years before and the image appeared to me in a moment of frustration. This image is part of a chain of associations.

The memory of my beloved dog represents a profound affective relationship that, though possibly regressive, was of the utmost importance to me here. It brought to mind the affectionate bond I had with my dog and the pain I experienced when he died, leaving a lasting feeling of absence.

In the chain of associations I remember other thoughts: this breed of dog is large and considerably strong, requiring attention by the person; they serve as personal protection and are loyal to only one owner; they are particularly good at promptly picking up on the owner's affective states when he meets a stranger, understanding whether the owner shows confidence and friendliness or uncertainty, suspicion and fear. The dog's behaviour will be different and adequate to his interpretation of the owner's non-verbal cues. The vigil alliance with the owner is founded on projective identification and on the sharing of feelings!

This insight was important because it allowed me to grasp the patient's hidden request and to develop my thinking.

This intuition and the subsequent associations made it possible for me to recognize Sara's profound and human need that came from behind her mask, and to connect it with my own feelings. The importance of my association was that it helped me understand my wish that there could be an atmosphere of profound affection, confidence and support in the analytic relationship as there had been with my dog, with the subsequent mourning of separation.

The second phase, characterized by the crisis of dissolution, abruptly shortened the emotional distance between the patient and me. Finally, Sara entered the analytic situation and came closer to the truth of the previously hidden unconscious aspects of her personality. She explicitly asked me for help, sharing the deep pain she had never previously consciously acknowledged nor revealed. Emerging from my own defensive position, I felt completely willing to start this therapeutic undertaking: a sort of first aid service (Alvarez, 1992).

I realize that many different and difficult factors may block the expression of feelings. In this case, I felt the need to provide 'first aid' when the patient started to manifest the anxiety of dissolution, the absence of bodily limits, the fear of losing herself and of having no shape.

I am aware that in such cases of disintegration the face of the analyst can be an important point of contact for the patient, but with Sara I offered the couch, first in order to restore the rules of the setting and to define our boundaries. Second, I also needed more distance than what was offered by the face-to-face position. I needed to be 'close to myself' and to think carefully about my own feelings. I feared that this patient tended to use her sight as a controlling mechanism and not as a way of thinking and communicating with words. She tended to use projective identification, and in return asked for symmetrical ideas or feelings from the analyst.

The patient reacted to the couch by revealing her secret pain and communicating the nameless terrors she felt deep inside. I hypothesized that she imagined she was a baby in a cradle on the couch instead of being an adult in front of me when we worked face to face.

So I maintained the relationship with Sara on two different tracks. Regarding the infantile part, I paid attention to the smallest bodily and verbal signs of communication. I left no space for silences, rather giving her ideas to reflect upon or memories of previous sessions that I associated with at that moment. During moments of serious dissolution, I provided a few words to sustain her. I did this as I felt she would become lost in the void if I left her with her own silences.

In terms of the more adult and basically omnipotent part, I listened, but did not interpret the content. I remained firm in maintaining the rules of the setting.

When Sara recalled dreams where she was unable to find a foothold in order not to be swept away by the current, she made me pay attention to the words, so that they could be something she could hold on to. Thus even here it was possible to develop feelings of empathy based on shared infantile experiences and on identification with the patient.

During this period, it was important to help her feel my presence, but with only a few words, to listen carefully to the communication and to share her difficult emotional states, sometimes only with a small vocal sound that meant I understood. It was important to ignore the late starts as well as disturbances from the outside, such as ringing telephones or meetings with other patients.

I tried to restrain my desire to provide interpretations and instead dealt with the part that was less recognized, far away from real feelings or thoughts, namely, the vacuum. It is important to offer a non-intrusive closeness, ready to give support when requested or needed.

As Tustin suggested during private supervisions (Tustin, 1980), in this period I agreed to answer questions regarding practical matters of life, especially on how to raise her son, who seemed to be in some danger; in fact, Sara identified entirely with her son rather than seeing him as a separate person with separate needs. I did not evade her questions or her doubts. When she asked me to explain something, I furnished explanations of a pedagogical nature, even though I knew the dangers of putting my analytic role to one side, but I was worried about her little boy. I subsequently verified that approaching Sara in this way and helping her to put sufficient trust in the analysis resulted in an abundance of dreams and also the acceptance of the rules of the setting. What these types of patients lack is the experience of frank interpersonal communication.

Once the analysis began, I prepared a welcoming environment, but in my mind I kept to the rules regarding the continuity and frequency of the scheduled sessions, as I have said previously. I made no analytic interpretations in this phase.

I considered that assuming an active role of containment and establishing limits was the only way to persuade Sara to follow me. She would quote whole sentences that I had previously said. She had written these down verbatim and kept them without processing them. Imitation is a primitive way of establishing a relationship, since introjection is still impossible. It is also true that one jots down notes in order to remember what one fears will be forgotten, whereas usually important things remain etched in our mind!

This position could be criticized, since it provides a situation that is overly agreeable or permissive and does not point out the hidden, manipulative and aggressive forces. However in my experience, in the absence of good internal objects, containment and the analyst's receptiveness are, in the long run, more fruitful than repeatedly clarifying the patient's aggressiveness.

The third period is characterized by Sara's realization of meanings that were different from those she had previously attributed (or did not) to past events. The transition to four sessions a week made it possible to speed up the analytic work and allowed me to intervene much more, since I saw her more frequently. Moreover, this rhythm stimulated Sara's attachment and the reflective function of that attachment (Fonagy, 1998).

It was important to repeat what Sara herself recounted. Giving a name to her feelings, and then listing a sequence of possible new meanings to her communications, provided her with new thoughts to take into consideration. By expanding the meanings in this way, she could try to broaden her way of thinking, thereby diminishing the omnipotence that had previously made her feel infallible and safe. Finally, after these processes, meanings could be linked together and the thoughts became more intense and complex.

All this, however, suddenly triggered the onset of ominous depressive feelings. These of course were at the opposite pole from her previous manic behaviour and made her think that the analysis was persecutory. She began to doubt the process, depression set in, she felt tired and thought she would seek refuge in a monastic lifestyle. Thinking at the cost of not enjoying herself in some hypothetical party represented for Sara a huge waste of time.

I then tried to show her that the absence of thoughts about the past was associated with the presence of pseudo-safety derived from a world of sensations and narcissistic defences. All her interpersonal affective relationships were at this time based on primitive, unprocessed, sensory experiences. She began to regard the results of the analytic work as being disastrous.

The interpretations, supported by the dream material and the material which now rose to the surface, were clear signs of what Resnik terms 'narcissistic depression' (Resnik, 1999, 2008). It was necessary to accompany her in this transformation and help her keep hope alive in order to find her own inner truth, thus suggesting a possible positive development in the future.

Moreover, it is important not to deflate the patient's narcissistic balloon too quickly, since the realization of her own failures could throw her into a vacuum of desolation or depression similar to that which had been experienced earlier in life.

Sara's further difficulty lay in the fact that her narcissism prevented her from reaching an actual depressive phase, which is necessary for the development of the undeveloped part of the personality.

Beneath an apparent normality that implies the existence of an object relationship, these adult patients hide a regressive part. Since projective identification is not used, this is then manifested in identity or somatic disorders. The deprived part does not communicate through projections in the normal way because it still has not reached the capacity of introjection, and needs to learn to receive and take in what is offered. If we do not create a way to listen to the non-being part, having clearly in mind where the patient's suffering is located, many classic interpretations are bound to end up in the bin or be nullified if the relationship comes to an end.

If we simply listen to the more structured part of the personality and respond to aggressive gestures, resulting in the patient's denial and mistrust, we trigger symmetrical responses, and the session turns into a minefield of misunderstandings and projections. Moreover, if we passively accept everything without intervening, we relinquish our therapeutic function altogether. We have to 'actively' wait for the real relationship to be established, and also accept the idea that we cannot be sure that our work will lead to a rapid and successful outcome.

We should also keep in mind that, even if the patient acquires greater cohesion and understanding of his or her inner world, they might bring back certain past behaviours as a weapon to destroy the analytic relationship and thus reclaim their freedom. The analyst who had fought hard to give more space to the conscious mind and promote more responsible behaviour finds herself having to point out previous repeated patterns, such as addictions.

Faced with the acting-out, I felt nullified and expelled from the analytic couple. At this point, I asked myself how I could reconcile letting the patient be free to choose and be responsible for her actions with the need for me to express my disagreements and the danger of her acting-out. I wondered how I could express my discomfort at her use of strength in acting on her instincts. Could my intervention again be felt as a judgement or an imposition, or was it useful as a way to represent a separation between us?

If I had merely listened to Sara's sadistic messages, she would have felt rejected by me, and would not have felt welcomed. Only when I was able to understand her emotional dearth could I transmit to her the passion and desire to work with her and help her: this is what she could then begin to feel, and this is what makes her return to the sessions. As I have recounted already, Sara had always reacted to real-life problems by saying: 'I'm leaving, they can all go to hell, they're all assholes!', as she did in her previous relationships; or she would pose threats: 'I'll commit suicide and thus take revenge on all those who misunderstood me.'

Over time, I came to understand that the phrase 'accepting the patient' takes on different meanings and possesses a different depth during different phases of the therapy. Initially, it means accepting the patient in his or her diversity, but also subsequently going over our own life experiences at the same time as those of the patient. It means understanding the characteristics of the patient's personality without resorting to our own preconceptions and judgements and without wishing for a speedy confirmation of our theories or psychological explanations.

It means being alive in the company of the other, or as Alvarez (1992) calls it, 'Live company'.

5.3 Reflections on the course of the analysis

The initial difficulty of giving a warm reception

At the beginning, it was difficult to accept Sara in my own mind because of the mask that concealed her confused identity. Through the transference, the patient projected onto me her unconscious tendency to separate her real affective life from the mask. This experience confirms that the Ego is committed to hiding the profound truth present inside each of us by means of language. I experienced my situation of discomfort as a block in the communication between my emotions, the world of my thoughts and my theoretical knowledge.

Sara's statement that she did not know what the word 'feelings' meant seemed strange to me after hearing so many accounts of her life, which seemed full of experiences. Sidney Klein (1980) says that these patients' feelings are flat. I would say that, in the relationship with Sara, the apparent feelings were friendly, but childish and volatile, they quickly vanished and were not in touch with profound emotions.

I believe that the inability of these patients to reach intense feelings is due to the difficulty of going through a process of symbolization and separation from an autistic state to a depressive phase and experiencing suffering from the loss.

Due to the difficult emotional contact and Sara's unusual attraction towards the exterior aspects of her surrounding environment, I gradually came to think that there was an autistic nucleus hidden behind her confused identity.

This initial experience confirms the hypothesis that the Ego, through language, is pledged to hide profound internal truth, as I have previously illustrated. As Groddeck (1929) suggests, language is confusing because communication reflects the misperception of internal life, and is directed solely by the Ego, which masks inner truth.

Only when I recognized Sara's hidden suffering, partly through physical signs, it was possible to establish an affective relationship. These signs then allowed the re-connection between my thoughts and feelings, and ushered in the affective relationship between us.

One could hypothesize here that the difficulty of recognizing Sara's primitive un-mentalized parts might explain the failure of her previous therapeutic attempts, which had lasted several years.

In reference to patients she calls 'normopaths' or 'disaffected', McDougall (1989) points out that the absence of affective contact in the relationship with the analyst is not due to an inability to express affective emotions, but to an inability to contain and intimately reflect an excess of painful affective experiences. Therefore, what is maintained is a detachment between emotions and their mental representations: I experienced this detachment during the first sessions, and this paralyzed my thinking.

McDougall makes analogous considerations regarding such patients who had to undergo many years of 'trial analysis' before getting closer to an affective internal world that had previously been un-representable.

This author relates an anecdote regarding the association of a patient of this type, who had refused at length to be helped and was verbally aggressive towards her. In reply to McDougall's remarks about his ambiguous relationship in the analytic context, he related this short story:

> Doberman dogs are considered to be unpredictable because of their personality disorder. One of these dogs was very fond of its owner and was able to transfer its love to a second owner, but when it was adopted by a third one, it tore him to pieces.

Realizing that her efforts in establishing a fruitful relationship with the patient were useless, McDougall was discouraged and asked him if she was his third analyst!

Bion (1959) helps us in our effort to come into contact with such patients. He believes that psychoanalysis is the practice of investigating mental processes and the internal workings of the mind, requiring constant observation. This analyst should not give in to an omnipotent desire to reach rapid and arbitrary conclusions.

The crisis of bodily dissolution and the role of the skin

The crisis of bodily dissolution heralded and highlighted a serious regressive state which led to Sara's dramatic loss of identity. At the time of the crisis, the sensation of no longer having continuity with her skin, which had disintegrated, made her feel that she had definitely lost her internal organs or, we might add, the internal objects associated with these organs. This made her lose the defences she had erected to fight against the terror of non-being.

As the vital importance of the sensory world diminished, a period of great confusion ensued in Sara and in her sense of Self. The loss of her encapsulated autistic refuge caused the loss of this former protection. This loss made Sara hypersensitive, as if she had actually lost the skin that contained her.

One of the first functions of the skin is to give the body a shape, to contain it, and to make it possible to perceive notions of inside and outside. In cases where the autistic experience prevails, the patient gradually realizes that the world of sensations has replaced the world of thoughts.

This lack of symbolization makes the body the only element that bears the truth, while the capacity of mentalization is too painful, and this suffering is evacuated as a bodily experience.

The following dream is in relation to the body and the skin:

> I am in Y, a place much higher than our country house, in a modest wooden cottage. I am with my mother and we find an impressive animal, small and triangle-shaped, maybe a crocodile, I don't remember ... it has no head and tiny legs at the four corners of its body. It has a shell, a kind of armour. The skin isn't like the skin of a crocodile, it's yellow and not green. We're afraid it's dangerous, because it has two pincers for legs. We catch it and put it in a transparent sack. I'm the one to capture it though it's slimy and transparent. It turns my stomach and makes me think that I've got to kill it. I take a knife and try to cut it in two but I don't have the nerve. Then I look at it and think 'poor thing', it might be harmless. It starts looking at me and is suddenly transformed into the face of a white cat, a kitten with pretty eyes, and so I say, 'oh, it's nice'. I pick it up, kiss it and cuddle it. My mother says 'be careful because you're allergic to cats', but I haven't had an allergic reaction for a long time. [She vigorously rubs her eyes at this point.] I've had other dreams like this, and like with the Rorschach test, you could interpret

them as having something to do with the idea of something not yet shaped, slimy. I think of abortions. I have a primitive perception of not being welcomed in my mother's belly. She always told me about her difficult contractions and all the problems she had when she was pregnant with me...

When I realize that the animal isn't dangerous, I start thinking: it moved quickly, darting like a lizard ... When I was 14, I was unhappy, my mother gave me a cat that didn't really interest me, it replaced my mother, it was a kind of substitute for her. Although I was indifferent to the cat, it loved me. After that, I started having allergic reactions.

In those days I managed to hold off my feline impulses.

The need to change one's skin

When Sara realized that she had built a false identity, she compared herself to snakes when they cast off their skin. She felt that she had to 'change her skin'.

Indeed, periodically, snakes shed the outer layer of skin. This is because their skin is not resilient and would not allow them to survive as their body becomes larger. Every time they shed their skin, it is replaced with a new one that is thinner and more fragile. It also seems that before shedding their skin they become irritable and stop eating! They hide because they feel vulnerable.

The mental development of human beings also requires changes in identity. Sara's analogy of feeling that she had to shed her own skin like the snakes makes one think that she could no longer tolerate being enclosed in an identity so rigid that it could not allow the act of thinking as a development of herself. This transformation required hard work.

Lack of symbolization of the concept of space

The process of symbolization that transforms physical absence into mental presence, and physical distance into psychic proximity is absent in this type of patient. An interpersonal relationship may be established by utilizing projective identification, thereby penetrating both the body and the mind of the other.

Sara did not seem to have developed the concept of three-dimensionality. Regarding autistic patients, Tustin (1986) compares the bodily image to a sheet of paper that has no inside or outside. Meltzer (1974) also takes up this concept and speaks of the two-dimensional nature of the autistic world (see Chapter 2, Section 2.8: Meltzer's 'two-dimensional world').

This lack of symbolization appeared during the sessions when, describing real or imaginary objects or persons, she had to repeatedly and carefully define their shape and size by gesticulating with her arms and hands in order visibly to convey the reality that she perceived. Mere words did not have the capacity or the power to communicate a mental representation. She thought that the listener would be unable to understand what she expressed, and the size and shape of the described object could only be demonstrated in a concrete way.

During the analysis, one of the most problematic concepts that emerged was the inability to symbolize the concepts of proximity and distance.

Once Sara became aware of her autistic withdrawal and her need to relinquish her pseudo-independence, she tried to imagine how to approach 'the other' in the analytic situation. Since proximity had previously been based on physical contact between skin and skin, resulting even in an imaginary state of fusion, a different space for communication in analysis now emerged.

Once Sara reached the stage of trusting, collaborating and feeling affection towards me, she thought she had come to such a stable situation that she could behave as she liked, as if the other would always be at her disposal, like an object she could just break or throw away as she wanted, without worrying about the other's feelings.

What the analyst needs to do here is to contain the damaged part and tolerate the inanimate part that the patient projects onto him or her. The subsequent step is to promote the process of separation by helping the patient reinforce her own identity.

Fear of attachment

In Sara's mind, the transition from affective indifference to an attempt to accept a tender relationship triggered the fear of attachment. These fears were expressed by memories and dreams relating to parasites. Sara was afraid that establishing a deeper attachment with me might make her claustrophobic. She was also afraid that I too might become so attached to her that I would grow tired of her and reject her. As she said: 'Patients who are seriously disturbed and are overly attached to their analyst end up tormenting her!'

She was afraid of becoming clingy, like parasitic insects that live on other animals or human beings. In fact, she found all such insects nauseating. She compared them to the close relationship between her mother and her sibling and to her need to feel attached to someone. The word parasite brought to mind a close physical relationship in which there was no request for help but rather a tyrannical control and an exploitation of the other. This concept comprises both the idea of a fixed relationship that ends by eliminating the parasite, as well as the idea of an adhesive one that does not envisage any space for communication. The concept of space between two people simply does not exist.

The matter of the parasites was also connected to the difficulty in asking for help, thereby relinquishing her narcissism. She told me about parasitic thoughts that invaded her mind, which she was unable to drive away.

Gender identification

Painful primitive experiences owing to the absence of maternal closeness, and subsequently owing to paternal disparagement and violence, had been encapsulated and pushed away. In order to maintain psychic survival, manic and narcissistic defences had built a misleading mask.

The female position was rejected because of this aforementioned early experience of not being in contact with an absent mother.

In her early adolescence, the structure of Sara's personality tended towards a male identification where the manic aspect prevailed along with omnipotence and narcissism. The father became her model, since he expressed vitality and strength despite his changeable mood and disparaging remarks.

The psychic collapse coincided with the experience of maternity as well as the cohabitation with her husband.

Sex addiction

McDougall (1982) used the term 'addiction' for a particular aspect of a solution that tends to disperse in different directions those emotional experiences that are too difficult to endure and differentiate. Resorting to some type of action (in this case, sexual acts) as a defence against psychic pain is a common practice during moments of stress, but if it becomes habitual it turns into an addictive solution.

In sex addiction, the dominant element is the fear of desolation, experienced as the death of the Self in the early stages of life. Sexual intercourse is imagined to be necessary in order to avoid the solitude and terror experienced in the archaic periods.

If people become abused themselves, instead of resorting to the use of substances such as alcohol, food, drugs or medicines, etc. as a panacea, they enter the category of Self-objects described by Kohut (1971), used as transitional objects.

The continual search for someone who would listen to her and welcome her with open arms and establish an imaginary fusion with her led to so-called 'feeling' relationships that confused her terribly. There was an absence of profound feelings and no thought that some meaning could be given to her relationships. The sensations inside her body gave her the idea of an inner life, and were mistaken for profound, lasting feelings.

The terror of emptiness and depressive feelings

The depressive feelings that appeared initially in Sara's analysis were expressed through bodily experiences of emptiness, inertia and weakness. They became manifest in the body as somatic disorders rather than being felt as psychic experiences. The lack of sufficient strength was also evident in her first dreams in which she wasn't strong enough to save herself from drowning. Sometimes the difficulty to come to her sessions was described as the absence of vital desire or a difficulty in moving her legs. These elements seem to refer to very early experiences of lacking support.

On the psychic side, at the start of the analysis, Sara proudly declared: 'I never feel guilty, I have no moral principles.' The analysis gave her a new vision of her past life, and provoked an upheaval of her identity. Many sessions took place in the midst of silent tears. At the time I interpreted these as an unspoken expression of the narcissistic wound, rather than a development towards a depressive position. She had tried many times to begin analytic work without reaching a fruitful understanding.

When I tried to stimulate new thoughts in Sara, instead of repeating the same fantasies, she suggested a 'new good idea', namely, having another child. I pointed out that in her phantasy the baby would fill her emptiness and thus relieve her from the effort of continuing the analysis.

As the analytic work developed, Sara pointed out that she had noted new thoughts in herself, but she knew they were not generated by herself as a sign of transformation. She hid the destructive feelings towards both herself and the analyst. A long time passed before I could interpret the transference and the content of her dreams. However, Sara gradually began to come to the scheduled sessions on time, which, in itself, testifies to a more solid affective involvement.

After missing a session because she had the flu, Sara returned with hypochondriac phantasies. She described this dream:

> I remember the dead child of a previous dream, perhaps it's a part of me that disappears. In front of the Monumental Cemetery there's a large open space near the gate. In the dream there are some marvellous small trees with delicate pink flowers like oleanders, just lying in their little pots on the packed earth. They have been brought there to be planted in the cemetery paths near the family plot where my grandmother is buried. The trees stay there for a few days since there are no gardeners to plant them out. There's a small hut that stores equipment and machines but nobody is there. I go to my assistants and order someone to plant the trees. I can't find anyone to do the job.

Sara makes the following association:

> I think the trees will be damaged if they are not planted in the ground. I feel the aesthetic need to brighten up the cemetery, or at least the small path leading to our family plot. The potted trees have to be planted without removing them from the pots.

I say that, faced with the discovery of events buried in her past, she would like to brighten up the cemetery with flowers that are new, fresh and cheerful (perhaps a new feminine nuance?). However, since the trees are in the pots and the roots cannot sink into the earth, they won't be in contact with the buried remains and they can't feed on minerals or water. The new parts cannot come into contact with the past and so be revitalized by them. It was hard to collect pieces of the past and build a personal history.

Once more, the aesthetic saves her from feeling pain. Sara recognizes that the aesthetic level perceived with the eye alone eliminates the pain, namely, her feelings. But she does not really understand what is meant by feelings. What this dream shows is the difficulty of helping this type of patient experience an affective contact.

Reiner (2012, p. 48) points out how:

> intersubjectivity reflects an intangible link between the two fields of interacting energies between patient and analyst. At the deepest level of the self, the heat created in primitive relationships provides the necessary energy that gives meaning and passion to the human experience.

What emerges in the process of Sara's analysis is the recognition of the lack of affectionate feelings, which are replaced by chronic rejection and aggression – feelings that provide a sense of individuality, strength and vitality.

The onset of these new feelings of affection for herself and for the other is an exciting experience both for the patient and for the analyst.

Note

1 The title of this section is what Tustin (1986) used to describe the bodily sensations of an autistic child. The use here of these two words is meant to acknowledge Tustin's creativity and confirm the feelings evoked when I found myself before Sara's crisis and pain.

References

Ackerman, N. (1938) 'The unity of the family', *Archives of Pediatrics*, 55, 51–62.
Alvarez, A. (1992) *Live company*, London and New York: Tavistock and Routledge.
Alvarez, A. (2012) *The thinking heart*, London: Routledge.
Bick, E. (1986) 'Further considerations on the function of the skin in early object relations', *British Journal of Psychotherapy*, 2(4), 292–301.
Bion, W. R. (1955) 'Language and the schizophrenic'. In M. Klein, P-Heimann and R. E. Money-Kyrle (eds), *New directions in psycho-analysis: the significance of infant conflict in the pattern of adult behaviour* (pp. 220–239), London: Tavistock Publications.
Bion, W. R. (1959) 'Attacks on linking'. In *Second thoughts: selected papers on psychoanalysis* (pp. 93–109), London: Heinemann, 1967.
Bion, W. R. (1961) *Experiences in groups*, London: Tavistock Publications.
Bion, W. R. (1962) *Learning from experience*, London: Basic Books.
Bion, W. R. (1967) *Second thoughts: selected papers on psychoanalysis*, London: Heinemann.
Cremerius, J. (1980) Personal supervision.
Fonagy, P. and Target, M. (2009) 'Mentalization and the changing aims of child psychoanalysis', *Psychoanalytic Dialogues*, 8(1), 87–114.
Freud, S. (1905) 'On psychotherapy', *S. E.* 7, 257–270.
Groddeck, G. (1929) *The unknown self*, London: C. W. Daniel.
Grotstein, J. S. (1990) 'Nothingness, meaninglessness, chaos and the "black hole"', *Contemporary Psychoanalysis*, 26, 257–290.
Klein, S. (1980) 'Autistic phenomena in neurotic patients', *International Journal of Psychoanalysis*, 61, 395–401.

Kohut, H. (1971) *The analysis of the self*, New York: International University Press.
Liberman, D., Grassano de Piccolo, E., Neborak de Dimant, S., Pistimer de Cortinas, L. and Roitmann de Woscoboinik, P. (1982) *Del cuerpo al simbolo*, Buenos Aires: Kargieman.
McDougall, J. (1982) *Theaters of the mind: illusion and truth on the psychoanalytic stage*, New York: Basic Books.
McDougall, J. (1989) *Theaters of the body*, London: Free Association Books Ltd.
Meltzer, D. (1974) 'Adhesive identification'. In A. Hahn (ed.), *Sincerity and other works: collected papers of Donald Meltzer* (pp. 335–350), London: Karnac, 1994.
Ogden, T. H. (1990) *The matrix of the mind*, New York: Jason Aronson, Rowman & Littlefield Publishers.
Ogden, T. H. (1992) *The primitive edge of experience*, London: Karnac.
Pichon-Rivière, E. (1971) 'Aspectos psicosomaticos de la dermatologia'. In J. Ulnik (ed.), *Skin in psychoanalysis*, London: Karnac, 2007.
Reiner, A. (2012) *Bion and being*, London: Karnac.
Resnik, S. (1999) *Personne et psychose*, Paris: Editions du Hublot.
Resnik, S. (2008) *Wounds, scars and memories*, Paris: Dunot.
Rosenfeld, D. (2006) *The soul, the mind and the psychoanalyst*, London: Karnac.
Schur, M. (1955) 'Comments on the metapsychology of somatization', *Psychiatric Study of the Child*, 10, 119–164.
Symington, N. (2002) *A pattern of madness*, London: Karnac.
Symington, N. (2007) *Becoming a person through psychoanalysis*, London: Karnac.
Tustin, F. (1972) *Autism and childhood psychosis*, London: Hogarth.
Tustin, F. (1980) 'Autistic objects', *International Review of Psycho-Analysis*, 7, 27–39.
Tustin, F. (1981) *Autistic states in children*, London: Routledge & Kegan Paul.
Tustin, F. (1984) 'Autistic shapes', *International Review of Psycho-Analysis*, 11, 279–290.
Tustin, F. (1986) *Autistic barriers in neurotic patients*, London: Karnac.
Tustin, F. (1990) *The protective shell in children and adults*, London: Karnac.
Ulnik, J. (2007) *Skin in psychoanalysis*, London: Karnac.
Winnicott, D. W. (1962) 'Ego integration in child development'. In *The maturational processes and the facilitating environment* (pp. 56–63), New York: International Universities Press, 1965.

Chapter 6

Irene
From robot-like to person

This chapter is the follow-up of a previously published case (Tremelloni, 2005), which is an example of a lengthy therapeutic journey from psychosis and autism to being alive in the world. It is here reconsidered as it pertains to skin in a psychotic episode of depersonalization. The deterioration of the skin expresses the terror of losing the integrity of the Self.

6.1 Case history

Irene's psychotic symptoms had begun with a crisis of depersonalization when she mistook the manic atmosphere of a discotheque for real-life hell. Initially, the gravity of Irene's situation was shown by the dramatic experience of not being able to distinguish living beings from dead people, as well as real people from the mannequins she saw in shop windows. She feared that if she shook hands with a person, that hand would be dead.

Another acute crisis was set off when a beauty treatment for acne caused a persistent redness of her face, which made her fear that her whole body and mind might be transformed and disintegrated.

In this case, as with Sara, the body's exterior, its surface and limits defined by the skin, together with external physical contact, had become of utmost importance.

It took her years to realize this when, seeing the wrinkles on her face, she became frightened at the changes in her skin and made a connection between her age and the time lost. She was also frightened because the position and shape of her wrinkles were not like the ones on my own face, which was another demonstration of a difference that impeded the process of identification.

When I met her initially, she seemed to be a psychotic patient. She possessed a marked paranoid state of mind, and had an imposing array of psychosomatic disorders (alternately, insomnia, hypersomnia, headache crises, sudden vomiting, anorexia and bulimia). Her body spoke in place of her psyche. The chronic recurrence of Irene's somatic disorders, which had resisted every therapeutic endeavour, conveyed the impossibility of finding comfort inside her mind, in the internal world of object relations. Even her verbal expression was limited; she also used some distorted words in dialect, which seemed to emphasize her inability to create links between words.

She could not obtain adequate answers in the grip of this primitive relationship, and this reinforced a phantasy of being excluded.

The in-depth analysis of our relationship clearly brought to light an autistic structure that prevented any kind of affective relationship. Irene's behaviour was so bizarre and rejecting that the answers she received from others were either a mirror that reflected her projected hatred or were incomprehensible. What ensued was a vicious cycle from which she could not escape. Irene suffered considerably inwardly, while outwardly she only displayed rejection. Her regular features and large blue eyes expressed bewilderment and anxiety.

She identified internally with a dead object. Her mother had often described her own repeated phantasies about the death of the foetus during her pregnancy with Irene.

6.2 The initial transference

Irene's psychic immobility and the prevalence of her persecutory thoughts made it particularly difficult to initiate and undertake analytic work. I repeatedly tried to find an explanation in the transference relationship, given that we had been meeting for such a long time, yet there were no apparent changes.

Her perseverance could be explained by her strong (though adhesive) attachment, sustained by crises of terror that ended in hospitalization.

I would like to highlight her rigid behaviour when entering and leaving my consulting room, in order to illustrate something about her participation in the analytic process. Irene would come in and leave with an evasive look on her face, saying 'good-bye' in a whisper, and with a detached manner designed to avoid moments of contact. She was mainly concerned about managing her bulky bags (autistic objects) that she brought in with her when she came into the consulting room. Recognizing the other became difficult when it was time to meet and to separate.

For years, she failed to acknowledge that our relationship was the result of any desire on her part; she saw it as almost mechanical. It seemed merely to give her the feeling of 'being in the presence' of a reassuring person that could listen to her. For her, the concept of time did not exist.

In fact, Irene felt the need to stay and work with the analyst in order to fill the emotional vacuum that she was not fully aware of. Her physical symptoms were the only evidence of this unexpressed need, and could not be healed by medical therapies. For example, a symptom such as sudden and uncontrollable vomiting would erupt in social situations, physically expressing contempt and hatred towards the outside world. This would make her presence disagreeable for everyone.

Once she got over the dissociative phase, paranoid ideation began to prevail, making interpersonal relationships very difficult. In the therapeutic relationship, the autistic experience prevailed. For a long time, it was impossible to interpret the transference. Although Irene was present, she was in effect not there.

In this connection, I recall Fairbairn (1940), talking about the borderline patient, saying that he finds himself repeatedly trapped in hating and being hated, while profoundly wanting to love and be loved.

The possibility for Irene to love or be loved was so distant that it was not discernible. She had been a seriously deprived child in a family environment that was both economically and culturally impoverished.

Alvarez (2012) points out that the feeling states of certain children may be so precociously frozen within themselves that there is not much love, not even hidden love.

Docker-Drysdale (1990) believes that certain children are unable to establish an object relationship, or they feel they do not need it. These children cannot symbolize what they have never experienced or been aware of.

6.3 Countertransference

As for me, in the countertransference, I shut myself up and remained passive, accepting Irene's bizarre behaviour during the sessions. I accepted her onslaughts and delays, her poor hygiene and neglect of her body, the predominance of her interest in serious physical disorders and the mental pseudo-deficiency that prevented her from making sense of everyday details in her life. I could not see how she might ever really benefit from therapy in the future. My bewilderment kept me from offering what I thought was some form of fruitful therapeutic help, while at the same time, I still remained interested in her confusion between life and death. Unlike the surrounding world, Irene found acceptance during the sessions; acceptance without rejection or judgements. Although I was irritated by her disturbing behaviour, I accepted her tenacious request for closeness as a decisive element, and carried on.

In my countertransference, I felt I was considered simply as an object in the room, and I was trapped in the situation of having to accept the absence of rules so as not to highlight her feelings of persecution. I did not know how long I could endure her abusive parts, however, or how beneficial our encounter would be. Nevertheless, I felt that Irene had the strength to cling to her therapy, without even knowing why.

Over time, my position of simply trying to contain her aggression and her bizarre behaviour brought about unimaginable changes. I think that my respect for her abused parts and Irene's own endurance of such abuse allowed her to relive the primitive phases of her affective development. During that time, I was always astonished by her bizarre and aggressive behaviour, and I simply 'waited in the wings' with no wishes or desires about our future.

I remained attached to the memory of my first encounter with Irene and her mother when she was hospitalized following her crises of dissociation. Although her anxious mother asked me to take care of Irene, it seemed to be more a request to become Irene's foster mother, because she herself did not know how to be a mother, but it was also an expression of love for her daughter. I have often thought back to this encounter: in that moment both had become my patients, in two different positions of suffering, in which I saw a difference. Although I have not seen Irene's mother since, the pain in this relationship has always been present in my mind, and this allowed their hatred and their need to be loved to be processed.

Our lengthy sessions demonstrate the extent of the confusion, Irene's need for attachment and her great tenacity in winning a place inside my mind, despite the persecutory phantasies and her initial negation of the interpersonal relationship. One could therefore only begin to imagine the extent of her primitive suffering and resultant autistic experiences.

6.4 Clinical course

For a long time, payment for the sessions seemed to be non-existent in her mind, since Irene did not know when the month ended and so she did not bring any money. Only after I asked for payment did she hand it over, on an unspecified day; it would be a crumpled cheque that she 'accidentally' found in her pocket. The transference should have made me experience at this time her profound sensation of being forgotten.

It took many years to introduce the concept of time and exchange, normalizing the act of payment, giving a meaning to her carelessness, and pointing out the denial of the relationship. She did not pay attention to her personal hygiene, as I have previously stated, and was shabbily dressed: she was in effect an uninhabited body. Her transformation came about very slowly as she began to have feelings of gratitude.

Once settled in the chair, she easily spoke, after many years of therapy, of her recent experiences, gradually giving her opinions and reflecting on herself rather than criticizing others. In the final years of the work, every time she related a gratifying achievement, she linked them with our previous conversations, thereby pointing out the changes that had taken place in her internal world as well as her gratitude.

After a few years of therapy, she started to study and obtained a diploma. Learning how to study was very difficult for her because she could not take in elements coming from outside. Studying was therefore a huge effort. She found it very hard to retain facts and to understand the meaning of words. Studying by rote (adhesiveness) was the only way she could learn, even though at the same time she realized that she was unable to understand the real meaning of the content.

One of the biggest problems came with learning a foreign language: she wanted to discover another way to express herself and to learn the meaning of the new words and sounds. But the difficulty of the process of symbolization blocked her efforts. Despite these problems, she attended free English courses in order to be better able to express herself.

She wanted to learn deaf-mute sign language, and she wondered whether such people had feelings and how they conveyed them. Another problem emerged when she started to learn how to use the computer. This became an endless persecutor when she made mistakes.

Although she continued having problems with real relationships in the surrounding environment, Irene always worked in a public health institution and was assigned various duties, including taking care of children or handicapped adults. She had a subordinate position and was under the control of supervisors.

Irene's long stays in various units were due to the fact that she managed to establish a relationship with the patients by identifying herself with the parts of the inmates that needed most attention. Without being able to limit the patients' countless requests, she earned their gratitude and, in this way, felt accepted. But in terms of the supervisors and those in charge, it was a different story. She refused to carry out their requests or advice, answered them in an impertinent manner or behaved so oddly towards them that day-to-day rapport became increasingly difficult.

At the same time, she always tried to participate in theatrical experiences as well as dancing school, to attend debates or social gatherings, but only in order to listen and improve her comprehension of facts and her integration with other people. This effort to change, in comparison with her culturally poor family environment, involved her increasing identification with me. Dedicating herself to her studies also represented an attempt to differentiate herself from her parents, from whom she had never managed to separate, neither physically nor psychologically.

She recently participated in a theatrical performance with a support group of people with Down's syndrome and other disabilities. The theme of the presentation regarded the behaviour of a group of robots that could only interact through numbers and mechanical hand movements. They were all dressed in white overalls that covered their heads and wore large pairs of striped glasses through which they could see but not be seen. They had a weapon to fight against monsters, and their bodies were hidden since they were all enclosed in a huge cardboard box that represented their castle. The final goal of the robots' repeated movements was to clean up the environment. They had to follow the commands that Irene gave them by calling out a number (human language had been replaced with numbers). A monster would approach and, out of fear, the robots would hurl their swords into the air. At this point, human beings arrived, removed the cardboard armour and the weapons, to uncover the head and face of the robots totally dressed in white. Thus each one regained his own human characteristics.

Irene comments:

> Initially, I didn't like this subject very much, but I later appreciated it because it made me remember how I felt in the past: it was as if I had been living inside an anonymous armour and I couldn't even show my body as a female, I felt protected by whatever clothing I came across; I didn't even

feel young and I thought I would live for eternity. I couldn't measure time or hours. I was not in contact with myself. I had no energy and I was weak. Now that I finally manage to see myself, I can think and express what I feel and think.

As she approached retirement age, Irene requested early retirement in order to take care of her parents, who were very old. Suddenly, there was an unexpected transformation. While in the past she used to have daily clashes with her parents, having never separated from them, now she felt a loving dedication, especially to her father. Every day she thought about where she could take him, where he could enjoy or distract himself. Irene was delighted to see how satisfied he was, and she took the trouble to satisfy his desires and look after his health.

Even her psychotic mother managed to change the way she interacted with her, transforming her desire to dominate her (which occurred with the same verbal violence and ferociously destructive criticism) into an attempt to provide understanding and accept her aggression and past weaknesses.

Irene's rage caused by the absence of welcoming, protective figures was transformed into respect and parental care. This brought about a change in the mother, who came to accept her daughter and her own dependence on her. For the first time, Irene experienced an inner fullness and well-being.

Along with all these transformations in the psychic area, some grave psychosomatic symptoms disappeared (migraine headaches, sudden vomiting, anorexia or bulimia) that had failed to respond to pharmacological treatment in the past.

6.5 Reflections

Irene maintained a therapeutic relationship with me from early adolescence right up to pensionable age, with a few interruptions in the first few years. This lengthy therapeutic relationship has given rise to many observations on my part about both the motives and the benefits that emerged during that time. It allowed changes to arise that determined the development of the Self. Certainly the initial psychotic symptomatology, underlying autism and overall picture of some form of real or assumed deficiency in states of mind did not forecast such a transformation.

The usefulness of the weekly sessions throughout her entire working life allowed her to discuss every sentence she uttered or every conflict that came up at the workplace. She needed an auxiliary Ego in order to help her have her own experiences. In this context, I always tried to point out the need to remain inside her own thoughts rather than fight against those of other people, paying the closest attention to my interpretations so that her persecutory fears, which would make her lose the trust that she demonstrated through her attachment to the therapy, would decrease. For my part, the position of containment of her aggression for such a long time made possible a succession of unimaginable transformations. I think that my respect for her abused parts allowed Irene to relive primitive phases of her affective development.

Irene internalized my capacity for containment that she had experienced during the analysis and managed to make a transformation. Recently (for the first time), she was able to create a phantasy in which she saw herself as a small light and gentle green leaf floating in a stream, probably in the spring. Although she did not know in what direction it was going or where it would arrive, it contained the idea of development over time.

After many years, she became emotional when she spoke nostalgically about the time that had gone by without her even noticing or knowing it. Once she visited a concentration camp and felt deep sorrow for those who had died there. For the first time, she cried during the session.

She was able to clearly describe not having been in contact with other people and with herself, and not knowing what 'feeling' meant. She explained that she had not understood that her anger was a feeling she transmitted to others. Previously, she had considered anger merely as 'an action to feel present and alive'.

6.6 Conclusions

After several years of being in contact with Irene, I continue to be amazed by the affection she shows me after all this time, and the awareness with which she is able to talk about her affective shortcomings remembering the total absence of feelings of the first years.

This case confirms Bion's hypothesis (1962) about the existence of preconceptions that can turn into thoughts only when such patients experience a human affective relationship that allows them this realization. Irene's determination and tenacity seemed instrumental in her search for something essential, even though she was unable either to think the thought or to express it.

One could say that, during Irene's long therapeutic journey, she was re-born, since she took possession of a Self that was able to create a relationship. She was finally able to realize that she had been living in a mental state that lacked a harmonious Self: she was now aware she had experienced fluctuations between being and non-being, living beyond time.

She now felt the pain she had endured, she recognized her story and the time that had passed with no thoughts. She perceived the absence of feelings in her previous relationships.

The change in the transference from start to finish was remarkable. From being unable to acknowledge others as living beings, establishing only cold and mechanical relationships, Irene was finally able to express herself, verbally acknowledging new situations and new feelings. In articulating her thoughts, she seemed to excuse herself for not having done so before, and she manifested her confidence in the fact that thoughts could develop within herself.

In his experience with mentally handicapped patients, Symington (2007) illustrated how psychoanalytic psychotherapy can help even in cases of 'so-called pseudo-deficiency' where the hatred of reality and new objects also generates hatred and rejection towards intelligence itself. Apart from the environmental, cultural and affective desert of Irene's experience with her parents, and her autistic withdrawal, the factor that contributed most to inhibiting her intelligence was a massive internalization of the maternal fantasies that were disparaging and destructive and the paternal affective absence.

According to Symington (op. cit.), the idea that one cannot work with persons with a low intelligence quotient is a false psychoanalytic myth. Perhaps the certainty of this idea can be sustained by the analyst's inability to get closer to her own mental handicaps. If the analyst cannot acknowledge her own omnipotence and subliminal contempt (which exists under the threshold of consciousness when one works with these patients), one cannot undertake the analytic work and think of the patient's psychic development.

I was surprised by the development over time of this patient's thought activity, and this led me to think about the unimaginable changes form the initial diagnosis. It is always inspiring to take part in those fortunate cases of transformation and acknowledgment of human values that had previously been buried or neglected and have now become a source of wealth.

Not acknowledging our contempt would make us fall into a trap: there is then a cycle of contempt-guilt-pity that hampers the analytic work. Pity does not allow the idea of development. If mentally handicapped people are treated in a protective and patronizing manner they cannot conceive of any possible change: they continue to remain in a passive and omnipotent position, used as a safe refuge.

References

Alvarez, A. (2012) *The thinking heart*, London and New York: Routledge.
Bion, W. R. (1962) 'A theory of thinking'. In *Second thoughts: selected papers of psychoanalysis* (pp. 110–199), New York: Jason Aronson, 1967.
Docker-Drysdale, B. (1990) *The provision of primary experience: Winnicottian work with children and adolescents*, London: Free Association Books.
Fairbairn, W. R. D. (1940) 'Schizoid factors in the personality'. In *Psychoanalytic studies of the personality* (pp. 137–151), London: Routledge and Kegan, 1952.
Symington, N. (2007) *Becoming a person*, London: Karnac.
Tremelloni, L. (2005) *Arctic spring: potential for growth in adults with psychosis and autism*, London: Karnac.

Chapter 7

Beatriz

Backwards love

This is the description of the analytic work with a suffering baby girl hidden within an adult woman.

During the process of analysis, Beatriz indicated that she had a personal dilemma regarding love and affective relationships. For Beatriz, the word love undergoes total transformation and the significance of the word is inverted.

Beatriz is a young, active and vivacious woman who brilliantly completed her studies, obtaining a Ph.D. in Physiology. At the age of 30, Beatriz began to suffer from optic neuritis and was very anxious that this was a symptom of a more serious neurological disease, like the one her maternal uncle suffered from. She also had a real loss of vision attributed to prolonged use of the microscope.

At the same time, she started having the first doubts that she was being persecuted by her colleagues: she started thinking that they had attached the squashed eyes of dead mice on her computer screen.

She worked in a laboratory where she treated genetically modified mice in order to study metabolic diseases. Beatriz was referred to me by a common acquaintance following hypochondriac phantasies regarding her eyes and persecutory ideation. In that moment, however, she refused pharmacological and psychological therapy because she had won a scholarship at a foreign university, and thus decided to move abroad. She had always dreamed of going away from her family in order to differentiate herself from them and become an important scientist.

After a short period of adaptation in the new job abroad, one day, without yet knowing the language sufficiently well, she left her apartment and wandered through the city with her computer. She entered a youth hostel and lay down on a bed without explaining what she wanted. So she was taken to a psychiatric hospital where the doctor diagnosed her with paranoid schizophrenia.

Leaving her family and her job and having to adjust to a new environment accelerated the outbreak of a psychotic crisis that everyone felt had come completely out of the blue.

The mask she wore to adapt to a normal life fell and the content of the delirium provided some truths regarding the patient's fundamental conflicts. The perception of the outside world became unreal and for several months prevented the patient from having a social life. The confusion regarding her identity unexpectedly appeared in the form of a dissociative episode.

No longer able to preserve 'normality' – at the cost of living an undesired life – the mask she willingly wore collapsed, and what emerged was her suffering. In the theatre of her own mind, she was the art director who needed to manipulate the other; as an actress, she performed a character in the play. She could not accept the fact that her structure had failed her during her crisis, and she was unable to acknowledge her depression and the profound narcissistic wound that prevented her from entering the depressive phase.

The start of delirious thoughts regarding her body began with the eyes. For a number of reasons, Beatriz connected sick or disturbing eyes with childhood memories or dreams. She saw the sadness in her mother's small and inattentive myopic eyes, which controlled interpersonal relationships instead of transmitting affection. Therefore, the fear of losing control through her eyesight brought out the difficulty of the interpersonal relationship with her mother.

Furthermore, during her childhood, Beatriz's mother worked in an institution that housed abandoned or disabled children. This may have exasperated Beatriz's feeling of being excluded by the mother, who spent more time looking after other children. Torn between a stormy relationship and the need of fusion, during the analysis Beatriz began to experience her mother's real illness in her own body, suffering from the same symptoms.

The body is given much attention as a place of primitive conflicts and confusion between one and the other. The concepts of proximity, distance, separation and individualization are not processed, such as, for example, the painful loss of the father who had died prematurely. Her phantasies about walking corpses bring back, in my opinion, the failed internal burial of the father, her only object of love and understanding. The experience of mourning probably led to a very destabilizing situation of affective vacuum: because of this danger, she unconsciously kept her real psychic reality at a distance until the moment she experienced a crisis.

The autistic nucleus came to light only during the analytic course where phantasies of lifeless and/or violent corpses, devoid of feelings, prevailed.

The lack of a supportive mother early on, and the loss of an affectionate fatherly support, led to the fragility of part of the Self. I thought that the voice of suffering had become petrified and thereby had always been removed from any internal dialogue.

Beatriz was the first of three children and had spent her childhood abroad in a modest yet problematic family environment: her parents were of different nationalities, her mother found it difficult to fit in and suffered from a depression brought on by illnesses and deaths in her own family, and finally, they had financial difficulties.

The prospects that her parents suggested regarding her future were grandiose compared to their economic condition, and Beatriz bought into them, even idealizing them. Beatriz interpreted the parental desire to improve the family's social and economic condition by attempting to achieve brilliant success in her academic career. From her mother's side, she assimilated the idea that a woman's success is reached only by marrying for economic advantage rather than for love. In order to make her internalized parents happy, she put herself to one side. Beatriz, however, became confused about what she desired in the relationships with the significant people in her life: she could fluctuate between unconditional possession of the mind of the other, idealized as true love; using the other as a support; or feeling contempt and rejection. In this way, the proximity or distance from others was more a displacement (attraction and rejection) of figures than relationships with persons who had their own feelings.

7.1 Transference

In the transference, there were attempts to ask for closeness and understanding, an expression of needy, infantile parts, which was often displaced by the need to assert herself as a powerful adult to be admired. However, the fluctuations in the countertransference made it difficult to perceive any continuity in the relationship and differentiate between the truth or formality of what she communicated.

Beatriz used a profuse array of language that tended to fill every space of our encounter, starting from the threshold of my study. The language was spontaneous, explosive and seemed to have the function of controlling my mind. One of her features was to describe in detail and irony facts or dreams, without actually communicating: in fact, any of my interpretations or comments on the content were challenged and rejected and considered ineffective or harmful. She couldn't bear silence, which she viewed as isolating, something that blocked communication. In this case, her words were autistic objects, used as protection against affective contact and actual communication of suffering. In this circumstance, the abundance and confusion of the topics made it difficult to find a common thread during the sessions, even though, through her words, dreams, thoughts and fantasies are expressed.

The difficulty in her affective relationships lay in the lack of continuity and duplicity of her feelings, which caused an uncertainty in her identity.

7.2 Countertransference

My countertransference went from recognizing that there was a real need for contact, demonstrated by the diligence and effort to stay in the analytic relationship, to feeling paralyzed in a vacuum with no real communication. The dependent and the bond were experienced alternatively with aggressiveness and irony or with the need to offer small, conciliatory gifts. Since the messages she had received from her psychotic mother were orders, signs of possession, contempt and criticism, the analyst's rules triggered reactions of rebellion and rejection. The only dependence Beatriz accepted was her addiction to cigarettes and food.

It is difficult to understand how to listen, how to make use of the material offered. The danger would be to remain fascinated by the creativity and strangeness of her stories and to stray from the search of hidden meanings.

In the absence of affective contact, her early physical experiences fostered phantasies regarding dead parts of herself, and transformed the bond of dependence into a mortal experience. Recurrent phantasies regarded suicides, homicides, corpses, gruesome crimes, poisoning. Instead of communicating and seeking help to emerge from her primitive suffering, Beatriz carried out a perverse transformation of her pain into a delirium, which she considered to be a work of art. The driving force of an imagined grandiosity fatally drove Beatriz into the world of mental disorder that carried with it a genuine fear of being no longer credible.

7.3 The truth in the delirium

The delirium represented a personal production that defined her, and in this delirium she felt she was someone who could think freely, without anyone imposing on her. Once the mask fell, the topics that emerged from the delirium were significant – unlike the patient's childhood experiences – and helped clarify her truth. They mainly concerned: the need to change the place where she lived (the family environment during her childhood was characterized by sadness, poverty, sickness, death); space-time disorientation (confusion of different periods, proximity, distance); maps of war strategies (how to defend herself); fearing someone would steal her personal data (control of her thoughts, penetration); doubts regarding gender identity (is there a gender identity that is more desirable?); the impression of seeing the surrounding real world backwards (wanting to change her personal story); confounding the personality of her family with that of unknown strangers (family members seen as strangers); the safety of having been adopted (refusal of being a descendant).

7.4 Clinical course

It seemed to me that Beatriz considered the analytic work less of an affective experience and more of a cultural one, even triggering literary ambitions; it was difficult for her to change her internalized relationships. Her delirious phantasies constituted the plot of detective stories that mingled violence and comedy, tragedy and desecration, terrorism and persecution. Writing represented the best guarantee that she knew of for thinking and knowing herself. In this way, the real suffering was nullified and shifted from the inside to the outside in her fictions. Violence, sadism, venom and the confusion between cradle and coffin were tempered by irony. What Beatriz needed was an audience that applauded her, recognized her worth and the exceptional nature of her thoughts. The only way to bring to life her deep-rooted story was to consider herself a literary work detached from her person.

Once she emerged from the acute crisis, the dream activities developed. But the numerous dreams did not stimulate any associations and were described like complicated news items. Since the connection between memory and emotions was painful, it was therefore eliminated.

The title of this chapter, 'Backwards love', derives from one of the patient's dreams based on a crime. The corpse of a man is found, a suspected homicide; nobody knows who the assassin is: as investigations are being conducted to find the culprit, guilt and accusations begin to circulate among family and acquaintances. In the end, the decision is that the culprit is the 'disaffection', that is, non-love, or better, backwards love: if one loves, one suffers; if one doesn't love, one is free from pain.

Gradually, a bond between us began to form after I accepted the instability of her feelings and the archaic aggressively that had been mitigated and transformed into irony.

The analytic work, which had begun following a moment of acute crisis, went on regularly and fruitfully for ten years, despite the difficulties in the patient's ability to listen. The analysis was interrupted by the patient, with the motivation that she had reached a notable improvement regarding her persecutory ideation and her level of integration. This was true in her social life: she had moved out and gone to live on her own in a new flat, she had taken exams and attended interviews for a new job, she began to earn a living, she wrote two historical books, winning a literary prize, and she consolidated her frequently unstable relationship with her boyfriend. Concluding our analytic work around the complexity of affective relationships may have caused her to be frightened about the possibility of experiencing desolation and primitive confusion.

7.5 Fairbairn's theory and Beatriz's psychic organization

Ronald D. Fairbairn's theory can shed some light on Beatriz's complex psychic structure. What follows is an outline of some aspects of Fairbairn's theory about primitive psychic experiences that can enlighten us in discussing Beatriz's clinical case.

Fairbairn (1940, 1941, 1943, 1944) introduced a new theoretical development of how the Self is formed, and his complex theory, at times difficult to understand, has been reassessed and further clarified by Ogden (2012).

Regarding the initial psychic experiences of the new-born, Fairbairn wonders whether early negative experiences can be attributed to a deficit in the mother's love of her infant or to the infant's misinterpretation of the mother's inevitable frustrations. Ogden holds that, according to Fairbairn's writings, one could assume that both conclusions are acceptable. The infant's total dependence, along with his need of total acceptance and help when faced with the experience of deprivation, makes him interpret any sort of frustration on the mother's part as a deliberate gesture of rejection. Every infant is able to detect the mother's limitations in her ability to meet his needs, and he interprets these shortcomings as her emotional refusal and lack of love.

When the infant experiences this deprivation, he will feel that his need for love is disregarded or belittled and his affective experience will be devastating. For an older child, the same experience will be the source of intense humiliation. When the deprivation is considerable, the infant will find himself in a state of 'worthlessness and destitution'. This sense of impotence will accentuate the notion that he is a bad child because he is being too demanding. At a deeper level, feeling unable and devoid of libido (nascent love) can bring about a sense of disintegration and imminent psychic death.

The threat of losing love – which is the only thing to bring the infant something good – triggers the terrible experience of losing a fundamental part of the Self, or even his own life. If, at a very early stage, the new-born experiences the lack of love that he needs, he feels he has destroyed the mother's love and that because his own love has been rejected, it must be destructive.

In that way, the infant internalizes the experiences of bad objects (which, according to Fairbairn 1943, are better than nothing since he cannot do without them!) and continually attempts to re-establish a loving bond even with an unloving or unaccepting mother. The infant's attempt to annul his own destructive actions in the bond and to gain – in vain – his mother's love can lead him to feelings of disconnectedness and death. In this effort to gain the unloving mother's love, he tries to survive by transforming the relationship with the external mother into an internal object relationship that becomes part of himself. If the relationship with the external mother is not satisfactory, the infant turns to this internal object that has become part of himself, thus alleviating the lack of love: both the real and the imagined unloving mother will be represented by an emotional vacuum.

The infant protects himself through the idea that his own mother feels he is unacceptable and projects these aspects in the relationship with unsatisfactory internal objects. These internal parts linked to rejecting or absent objects elicit negative emotions, which are repressed, and there is a continual effort to change unsatisfactory objects into satisfactory ones. Fairbairn considers that the internal objects are 'not just objects' but are dynamic structures that interact with other structures more or less capable of primitive psychological activities.

Fairbairn hypothesizes that the infant divides the internal object (the unloving mother) into two parts: one is alluring and the other rejecting. One aspect of the infant's personality is strongly attached to the alluring aspect of the internal-object mother, while the other part feels attached to the rejecting and hopeless internal object. According to Fairbairn, through successive projections of the Ego, identification with the different parts of the internal objects creates different unconscious relationships between a tantalizing Self and a Self that identifies with the exciting object, and between a rejected Self and a Self that identifies with a rejecting object. These sets of relationships between internal objects represent different relationships between aspects of the Ego.

The love and hate that unites internal objects is in this case pathological because it is derived from the infant's pathological bond to an inaccessible mother felt to be incapable of giving and receiving love. Therefore, what is established is a relationship between the libidinal Ego and the exciting object – which Fairbairn terms 'addictive love' – due to a desperate need of the exciting object to trigger the desire of the libidinal Ego.

Fairbairn has pointed out that some patients find it difficult to relinquish pathological attachment to unconscious relationships with internal objects. This attachment arises from the constant need to transform bad internal objects into a type of person that would be desirable to have as an object.

In conclusion, referring once again to Fairbairn's theory, the internalized and interconnected primitive relationships are at the root of adult affective relationships. One thing alternates with another: the need for love, in which one cannot really believe; the excitement provoked by the other and the desire to love and be loved; the need to identify with the rejecting object and with the self-rejection that is full of hate towards the unaccepting mother. Stable affective relationships have become impossible and are regarded as prisons or illusions.

References

Fairbairn, W. R. D. (1940) 'Schizoid factors in the personality'. In *Psychoanalytic studies of the personality* (pp. 3–27), London: Tavistock/Routledge & Kegan Paul, 1952.

Fairbairn, W. R. D. (1941) 'A revised psychopathology of the psychoses and psychoneuroses'. In *Psychoanalytic studies of the personality* (pp. 28–58), London: Routledge & Kegan Paul, 1952.

Fairbairn, W. R. D. (1943) 'Phantasy and internal objects'. In *The Freud-Klein controversies 1941–45*, London: Routledge.

Fairbairn, W. R. D. (1944) 'Endopsychic structure considered in terms of object relationships'. In *Psychoanalytic studies of personality* (pp. 82–136), London: Tavistock/Routledge & Kegan Paul, 1952.

Ogden, T. H. (2012) *Creative readings: essays on seminal analytic works*, London: Routledge.

Chapter 8

Monica
The psychic retreat

In the case I am about to describe, the existence of autistic residues was evident from the first moment, and had been identified by the patient herself as the source of her relationship problems. The countertransference was very difficult to deal with because along with a request to be helped came an inability to change and a continuous refusal of emotional bonds with others.

Monica was a pleasant woman in her forties, with a bright yet static face and no sign of femininity in her attire. At the beginning of our sessions, after having muttered some things under her breath about the weather or some such thing, she would put on some lip balm, as one does to protect lips from cold or windy weather. Could speaking be dangerous?

She talked about her problems with determined and precise language, and I immediately sensed that she held much hope that she might be listened to and understood, yet she had no desire to listen herself.

After graduating from university, Monica began to deal with political and social issues. She was married and had three children. She was aware of her emotional difficulties and had already had therapeutic interventions in the past, but at the time of our meeting she was overcome with preoccupations regarding her inability to raise her children and feel like a mother.

8.1 Clinical course

Upon accepting the patient, I felt like I would be able to understand what she consciously brought to the session; at the same time, I was also aware of a defensive part, the part that was unknown to her. Though in our contact I felt like an outsider, it also seemed that the patient was in some way secretly acknowledging the offer of my presence and understanding by agreeing to carry on with our sessions. The continuity of physical presence in our sessions, however, did not correspond to any emotional closeness.

Monica showed no signs of natural empathy or wish for empathy from another person; she seemed to only wish for someone who would listen to her, and – simultaneously – who she could dominate and belittle.

Monica's behaviour did not take others into account, and in speaking of her childhood, she reported feelings of rejection or degradation, and a general awareness that she had not been acknowledged as a subject; she complained of serious difficulties in establishing emotional contact and spoke of problems in social relations as an adult. Her professional life was marked by insecurity and lack of creativity, despite the fact that her family was culturally stimulating and had passed on a facilitating model. Her emotional disorder had also damaged Ego development and symbolization, resulting in dearth of thought. She could not stick to a schedule and there were frequent errors and omissions. The language of affection was missing, and hard to learn. Nonetheless, Monica appeared to lead a 'normal' life, managing family and work commitments.

Monica continued her analysis but remained non-empathic: she displayed a dominant attitude of rebuff and pessimism, and did not budge in her critical and deprecating stance about every interpretation or intervention I made. Her speech was fluent, but the volume of her voice changed easily from high to an almost unintelligible low, and this represented, in my opinion, an attempt to come closer to me, followed by her pulling away. Her tone, on the other hand, affirmed the unchanging nature of the content of her speech. Her accounts of daily events tended to focus on negative experiences. Any reference she made to the fact that she lacked feelings and was unable to change seemed to be absolute and not questionable.

Symington (2002, p. 187) refers to these absolutes as 'godlike', as though they were of divine origin and therefore not open to rational discussion: the more jelly-like and insubstantial the internal state, the more petrified and 'godlike' the external solemn statements.

Monica declared almost proudly that she had no feelings towards anyone, and least of all for her family members. This was, in her opinion, an unchangeable characteristic, justified by her primitive feelings of frustration. In my opinion, her discontent regarding her lack of feelings was only superficial: there was no real sadness about this because her hardness towards others represented the only strength of her personality. She would inexorably come back to the description of the humiliations she had endured, which, according to her, had been inflicted on her by every member of her family. While acknowledging that the past could not be changed, she would not accept the possibility of changing her present assessment regarding her internal objects. Monica carried the notion that contact was impossible into the analytic relationship as well as into her everyday life.

We can consider this to be a form of addiction to a past that is very close to psychic death. Her outer mask appeared childish when compared to her actual age. It was as if she wanted to maintain the mental state of a child.

8.2 Transference and countertransference

Monica occasionally spoke of ending her analysis, thus exhibiting her power over me; the fact that she continued seeing me for several years seemed to be more owing to her difficulty in separating than to her awareness and expression of an actual need.

I wondered what the motives were, both for the patient and for myself, in continuing the relationship, since there was no change in thinking. I had several hypotheses: for example, I thought that analysis might represent for Monica a sort of permanent identification with her internalized and rejecting parents, and that her unconscious purpose was to make the analyst experience and understand her suffering by deprecating and immobilizing me, making me feel just as she had felt: a sort of unconscious, acted-out revenge. It could also be an expression of the difficulty in differentiating attachment from hatred. Or perhaps it was a way of maintaining an ideal attachment in the sessions by trying to transform – through physical presence – affective experiences into concrete representations, as is done in theatre performances.

I thought that her perseverance could also represent a way to challenge the analyst, like a showdown to see how long I would remain present and accepting in spite of her effort to make me analytically powerless. It could also indicate the need to experience long-term loving and nurturing care, or to secure a life insurance against the risk of being alone. In any case, her narcissistic barrier did not permit any form of listening, nor any change of thought. All this made creative processes difficult, including in her professional work. She seemed to want to take any hope for change away from me.

As for me, I sometimes felt discouraged or irritated at not being acknowledged as an ally and innovator, and for being mocked in my effort to understand her. At the same time, I sensed the presence of a state of suffering and deep solitude within the patient, who was subjected to internal trials that were difficult to overcome. Steiner's concept of psychic retreat (1990, 1993) was illuminating in this therapeutic relationship.

I often wondered how to proceed, given the static nature of the analytic relationship, the boredom brought on by the repetition of the same themes and behaviours, and the irritation that came from her continuous deprecating and sadistic attacks. To suggest ending the analysis because of a lack of change would have represented a further and unequivocal refusal of the patient by the analyst/parent. Furthermore, it could have meant the destruction of any hidden hopes for the future. Should I settle for her efforts to maintain her professional and family relationships within acceptable boundaries? Or should I accept the failure of the analysis, labelling it as one of those un-analysable cases, so that I might feel less incompetent? My fantasies went from acknowledging my masochistic tendency to withstand denigration, to a sense of professional responsibility, to my concern for the patient's emotional fragility and emptiness of thought.

On the other hand, the questions Monica raised about the mother/children relationship (past and present) elicited in me fluctuating thoughts and a strong interest regarding the role of the woman. My only attempt was to highlight her new efforts and connect these to the encouraging responses she received from others.

At the beginning of this therapy, I felt a sense of solidarity with Monica in listening to the events of her life, and despite her difficulty in asking for real help, I sensed her need for a supportive alliance. Over time, however, my affective empathy started to fluctuate negatively. The only way to restore positive empathy and continue the relationship was for me to think about her story, her past and present, and to process my countertransference rigorously.

Aragno (2008) differentiates between ordinary empathy, which is usually immediate, and empathy that lasts over time. Goldberg (2015) also makes a distinction between these two types of empathy, stating that they are different not only in quantity, but also in quality: to maintain empathy through time, the analyst must make an effort to continuously adapt internally, so that she or he may be able to share different feelings. Time provides explanations; it historicizes connected facts and feelings and offers different perspectives and interpretations. One of the difficulties the analyst faces in therapies that last over long periods of time is keeping the 'enduring empathy' alive and balanced.

I was thus making attempts to escape boredom, depression, rejection and the idea of failure, trying to find possible similarities between Monica's painful experiences and my own in order to come closer to her state of mind and avoid distancing myself or taking on a judgemental attitude. These efforts offered no evident results in the development of our relationship, though they did bring about some improvement in her work and in her professional relationships. Nevertheless, I kept hoping for a change in the patient's mental state. All this led to very intense work in my emotional world so that I could be able to tolerate that which was different from me and to search for new ways to communicate.

In addition to patiently waiting for change, I believe that in these cases one must also exercise caution when intervening with words. One needs to be mindful of when and if certain assumptions or observations should be communicated to the patient, and if these could potentially be hurtful or written off, thus blocking any further listening.

When we talked about feelings, Monica often used the word 'formal' to mean that, in communications between one another, feelings can only be stated by social convention and do not correspond to 'a real feeling in the body'. In Monica's case, the dissociation from emotions transformed feelings into words that contained nauseating, despicable and false elements.

8.3 Conclusion

The turning point in which the patient went from being distant and disparaging to being more empathic took place when we met after yet another tragic occurrence in Monica's life.

After hearing what had occurred, Monica saw in my expression a spontaneous sign of emotion. She could see the physical and tangible sign of my emotional closeness 'with her own eyes', unlike my empathy of the past years of analysis, which she could neither 'feel' nor acknowledge with her mind. In fact, in the dialectic of her internal world, she could neither believe in nor experience a sincere alliance.

Finally, the visual perception of shared feelings in a moment of severe psychic pain allowed for new developments in her thinking, enabling the analytic relationship to unfold. The new trauma unexpectedly led to some form of processing, and Monica was finally able to use emotional nuances in her statements and listen to my words. From a statuesque stillness, her face began to show movements and expressions, and the tone of her voice became less harsh.

A long period of time was necessary to get over the severity of the trauma, and at that moment, her feelings were once again at the centre of our conversations but had become more truthful or more alive.

A more creative dynamic was finally beginning to take place, though it was still too difficult to express emotions directly through words. The fact that she started bringing me an occasional flower, picked in the garden, showed that some change had taken place. I thought, upon accepting these flowers, that this was a concrete relational gesture, and perhaps the beginning of a process of acknowledgement that could take place without being translated into words. When Monica began to talk about the end of her analysis and express her concerns about how she would face the difficulties of the world on her own, she offered me a plant that she had specifically chosen – she told me – for the scent of the flowers and the strength of the species, suggesting that I could plant it on my balcony. I pointed out that the roots planted in my soil represented her desire to remain close to me in my mind, and the plant's growth and new shoots were linked to her future development.

When I heard in Monica's voice and words a new feeling of emotional contact and recognition – after such a long period of her denying all feelings – I was overcome with emotion. This created a situation of 'complex understanding' which encompassed the sharing of all the real trauma of Monica's life, the difficulties of our analytic encounter, the nostalgia for the time spent together and a stimulating sense of hope and satisfaction. Only at that time could Monica admit to feeling pain about our upcoming separation, saying that she did not know how to think about it or approach it because it was something new in her mind, something she had never experienced before.

My initial interest in this woman who was seriously struggling yet unable to ask for help was the driving force in the development of the analysis.

Every analyst has a hypothesis regarding what brings about the patient's change in state of mind, which heralds the conclusion of the analytic work and differs in each case. If the patient's thought fails to evolve, one must abandon the original therapeutic project, and in order to continue the therapist must reconsider previous hypotheses and known theories, experience a real possibility of failure, and accept what the patient is able to feed back. Every attempt to connect with one's own feelings may be followed by denial, and only patience, constant self-analysis and the analyst's hope for the future can allow the relationship to continue despite these difficulties.

In these cases, where there have been so many years of denial of the passage of time, we must consider that a new vision of oneself and of personal time may lead to states of disappointment and depression, which differ from previous depressive states: this new state is more vital and connected to the novelty of feeling.

Retrospectively, I think that the time and effort required in maintaining a sufficient degree of empathy have been proportional to the severity of the patient's illness and to how early on the initial trauma occurred. In the end, the time and effort brought about the possibility of 'feeling' and living a life with some hope for love.

I'd like to conclude by saying that these long and difficult analytic trajectories help the analyst undergo continuous internal transformations, for which we must be grateful to the patient who – for a certain period of our lives – accompanies us in our life journey.

8.4 Steiner's psychic retreat and Monica's resistance to change

The term 'psychic retreat' (Steiner, 1990, 1993) refers to a defensive reaction in the pathological organization of the personality of neurotic, psychotic or borderline patients: when faced with unbearable anxiety, the reaction is to find relief by retreating into a sheltered space. This area represents a safe haven; the pathological organization acts as a delicate system of defence by which the patient maintains his or her paranoid or depressive anxieties.

Steiner believes that these states are experienced as if they were places where the patient can find peace and escape from the unbearable anxiety of coming into contact with others. The retreat might serve to control primitive destructiveness, and represents both a receptacle of destructiveness and a defence against it. Because it is a kind of compromise, it is pathological, but it provides an area of temporary protection and isolation from contact with reality. On one hand, it protects the patient, while on the other it represents an obstacle to the patient's development.

The area of psychic retreat hampers psychoanalytic work from developing and the therapist must practice patience and perseverance to alleviate the pressure put on by the patient and understand the defensive organization. Treating a patient such as this is difficult since she or he is not in contact and, consequently, the analysis progresses very slowly.

References

Aragno, A. (2008) 'The language of empathy: an analysis of its constitution, development and role in psychoanalytic listening', *Journal of the American Psychoanalytic Association*, 56, 713–740.

Goldberg, A. (2015) *The brain, the mind and the self*, London: Routledge.

Steiner, J. (1990) 'The retreat from truth to omnipotence in Sophocles' Oedipus at Colonus', *International Review of Psycho-Analysis*, 17, 227–237.

Steiner, J. (1993) *Psychic retreats*, London: Routledge.

Symington, N. (2002) *A pattern of madness*, London: Karnac.

Part III

Chapter 9

First encounters
Adventures into the unknown

> ... we were so close to the coast that we could make out various people on the beach who seemed to be of a dark or black colour, but who we could not distinguish from the clothes they were wearing.
>
> (James Cook, 22 April, 1770)

Naval officer James Cook (1728–1779) was sent on a mission by the British Crown as commander of the vessel *Endeavour* (1768) to conduct astronomical and geographical investigations. He was to observe – from a certain point of the Earth – Venus passing in front of the sun, and discover a supposed continent called Terra Australis Incognita. Cook was chosen because of his expertise in mathematics, cartography and astronomy, skills that led to important discoveries in scientific and geographic fields.

In the travel journal taken on one of his trips, in April of 1770, he describes the first encounters with the indigenous peoples observed from the ship, a short distance from land: these men appeared to him to be different from the men he had known up until that point; he first describes their size and the colour of their skin, which looked like 'the colour of wood or chocolate'. He could not distinguish clearly whether the colour was of their skin or of the clothes they were wearing. He differentiated these individuals from Africans because of the differences in hair: one type was unkempt and thick, the other thin and with small curls. The physical differences of these inhabitants signalled that these lands were different from the others he had already encountered.

Cook undertook three voyages, probing the Atlantic and Pacific Oceans. The third voyage (1776) was intended to discover the fabled Northwest Passage. On his way to the American Northwest, he ran into the Hawaiian Islands.

From the descriptions of the first encounters, it appears there were attempts, by both parties, to come into contact with the stranger, offering gifts or hospitality, which were answered with, alternately, curiosity, rejection, distrust and aggression. The British crew could hear the sounds of an unknown language and could only understand the meaning of a few words through movements and facial expressions when they had to communicate a need, for example, to stock up on water or firewood. Mutual curiosity was associated with fear, and the exchanges took on alternating forms.

The arrival of Cook's ships in the Hawaiian Islands coincided with some indigenous religious rites, and was therefore laden with meaning in that it led to Cook being personified as an important Hawaiian god, Lono. This contributed to his deification and, thus, to his acceptance. However, differences subsequently arose between the natives and the British about material stolen from the ships, which was initially of little significance, but then grew and led to the killing of Cook during his third trip (1779). Both the natives and the English crew demanded to keep Cook's body, so that his bones were divided up amongst the contenders as a sign of the particular emotional significance invested in his person.

The encounter with never-before-seen people stirred in both parties a set of mixed feelings that made it difficult to understand each other's less explicit intentions and build productive relationships.

In the analytic encounter, the manifest intention of both parties is apparently clear and defined, although in reality the patient's request contains many unknowns, many contradictions, illusions and fears. We ourselves do not know initially if we will be able to establish a therapeutic and satisfying relationship. Any encounter with the unknown can be exciting for us all, as it represents the beginning of an adventure of which we do not know the duration, the way it will develop or the emotions it will arouse.

From the observer's point of view, an important element in providing an attentive and welcoming stance towards another person is given by the state of mind. There may be differences in the personality of the therapist: natural empathy, different theoretical positions or the mood of the moment.

In any case, knowledge about the other is first gained through our physicality, our body and our senses, in particular through our sight and the signs from the other's body. Finally, we obtain more refined elements of knowledge through our hearing, by listening to the language. The immediacy of the observation provides us with many important elements: age, figure, body shape, gender, face, words, way of speaking and movement. We see these objective elements and, at the same time, we submit them to our own way of interpretation. What is expressed through the body and the word is interpreted in a personal and arbitrary way to build a working hypothesis. Is this already a 'psychoanalytic' observation?

Resnik holds that the task of the 'analyst-archaeologist' is to observe, describe and interpret the elements that have remained buried in the unconscious, elements that come to light through symptoms and signs (Resnik, 1999).

It can be said that transference starts as early as the initial observation, and the analyst seeks to transform perceived concrete phenomena into a possible dialogue.

The impression that is most significant to us is the perception of the face, which is a synthesis of the history of the past and the present. The face, and in particular the skin that covers it, summarizes the person's life experience and manifests the traces of their labour over the years, their history, and the presence or absence of a thought activity (Resnik, 2008). Specifically, the skin that covers the face shows signs regarding the state of the subject's health and his or her actual or manifest age.

Moreover, the gaze and eye contact seem to give a better understanding of the other's state of being. A look into the other's eyes, in addition to picking up aesthetic characteristics, can have the intention of penetrating the personality (an intrusive gaze) and taking possession of the other's most secret sentiments. If insistent, the gaze may constitute a transgression of the other's intimacy.

In autistic children, the avoidance of eye contact makes the other non-existent and is a way to avoid personal contact; it is part of the wall erected to protect from the non-Self of the outside world.

In a split-second, sight summarizes the 'person' as a whole and leads to fantasies or associations with other personal elements that come to mind. In this case, the sense of sight leads the discriminatory and complicated activity of thought.

Hearing, too, will provide us with important information about the other, through tone (mood), volume (aggressiveness or penetrative intent), changes in voice level (emotional fluctuations), the speed in which words are formulated (possible greed) or – finally – silence (sometimes as the negation of contact). These variants are connected to unconscious experiences of a pre-verbal period.

Language in general conveys important messages that are decoded over time. In reproducing a conversation with her mother, a patient spoke with a shrill and intrusive tone, an expression of the level of hatred and rejection she experienced in their relationship, and then placed in the transference. This happened because it was impossible for her to express it symbolically through words, and so the feeling of aggression in that moment was not recognized as something personal. We can grasp its relational meaning through our feeling of acoustic discomfort and through our associations.

Another element of attention is the other's age, which is found in a temporal relationship, relative to our life and age. Generational differences may emerge, or identifications in the same age group of the observed. A few decades ago, ripped trousers were a sign of the individual's poverty and difficult conditions. I wonder what they mean today: a mask for the rich or the expression of a rebellion against conformism, or perhaps just a replica of a social model different from the past? The observer thus makes personal associations to his relationship with the environment and the experiences of his lifetime. We must not forget the importance of external appearance, given by clothes or make-up or hairstyle, which falls within the construction of 'the mask'.

Similarly, the subject will also suggest different associations for the observer. The psychotic patient may present behaviour or verbal expressions that may seem incomprehensible or bizarre: only a prolonged period of observation will allow us to look for the hidden meanings of such communications.

One may perceive diverging intentionalities between physical expressions and verbal expressions, or the dissociation of the 'physical I' and the 'psychic I' as two separate entities. The analyst tries to formulate a personal portrait of his/her patient in an arbitrary manner by using the information reported, the hypothetical meanings of body language, and by trusting the emotions arising from his unconscious. These are primitive and confused emotions that need to be recognized and differentiated. In the end, all this information will be processed and will form a storyline on which to develop (or not) the analytic relationship.

Meltzer (1968) imagines that, when we meet a person in a situation as significant as the analytic one, our unconscious constructs a dream and places the other within it, in a role that is assigned to him by our world of emotional experiences. So, the other comes into the intimacy of our life and, depending on personal developments and the experience of the encounter, his role can be changed repeatedly. Thus begins an imaginary coexistence: in fortunate instances, that of a fertile exchange, a new story, written by both, will be born. Otherwise, the fixed nature of the roles will prevent the development of the relationship and will foster the repetition of the past. In the countertransference, we experience the ups and downs of this imaginary internal coexistence, which will accompany us during the analytic work.

The information given by our conscious mind can be in agreement or in stark contrast to that provided by the unconscious part of our mind. What corresponds to the patient's truth and what corresponds to the mask? And, if the information is in contrast, how can it be reconciled in our minds at the beginning of the relationship? The possibility of immediate error can be due to the presence of a false Self that cleverly masks the true Self.

In the case of adult patients with autistic mental states, what initially appears may vary, depending on the individual defensive constructions, and these can simulate a Self that has accumulated certainties and skills. The deficient area of affections remains to be discovered. The transformation of the false Self into the true Self, through analysis, becomes long and difficult. A prolonged observation and the processing of our countertransference will help us see what was invisible, put all the data together and interpret it.

References

Meltzer, D. (1968) 'An interruption technique for the analytic impasse'. In A. Hahn (ed.), *Sincerity and other works: collected papers of Donald Meltzer* (pp. 152–165), London: Karnac, 1994.
Resnik, S. (1999) *Temps des glaciations*, Ramonville-Saint-Agnes: Eres.
Resnik, S. (2008) *Wounds, scars and memories*, Paris: Dunot.

Chapter 10

Transference and countertransference

10.1 Transference in patients with autistic experiences

This topic has already been discussed in the first part of the book. I will add a few more general considerations here.

Transference and countertransference are part of a mutual dialogue in which thoughts and feelings are shared. Communication can take place only if the other's 'otherness' is respected by both participants; however, when there is poor integration of the patient's personality, communication does not always happen symbolically. For this reason, the analyst must initially adapt to staying in the realm of the concrete, and then help the patient bring symbolic meanings into communication with 'the other'.

Susan Isaacs (1952) associates the transference situation with a mental construction based on primitive experiences, and so with a set of unconscious phantasies that can be thought of for the first time as emotions of the past after a great deal of work. In the past, these emotions had arisen too early and were therefore too disturbing to be experienced, acknowledged and translated into language. In transference, feelings of love and hate reappear towards the therapist as a representative of the patient's parents. Transference, through resistance, contains the ambiguity or confusion of conflicting feelings. In psychoanalytic practice, a space and a time to meet are defined, but in the interpersonal relationship, the past becomes present.

If initially, in acute situations of disintegration, transference conveys a need for fusion of bodies and a confusion regarding limits, later, having reached a further stage in which interpretative work can be introduced, the patient's primitive attitude can change suddenly. It can be replaced by attempts at manipulation that aim to transform the analyst in order to fit the patient's own design. In these cases, the transference can bring to light confusing messages that come from the patient's dissociated parts.

The analyst initially notices a distance in the interpersonal emotional relationship, where feelings of alliance are normally intertwined, with a common purpose in view. The patient's usual defensive mode is re-activated and intense projections prevail, disturbing the analyst's evenly hovering attention. These projections are irritating for the analyst as they limit his or her freedom to think. The analyst may feel depressed due to the continuous attacks and undermining tactics; he or she may become bored by the repetition of the same defence mechanisms and the constant manipulation, and may have fantasies about expelling the patient or responding through actings-out of her or his own.

When the relationship with the analyst is adhesive, the patient may be interested in the analyst's body, clothing and perfume, and may be curious about his or her private life. He may show a lack of respect by being constantly late to the sessions or in making payments on time.

Often, the transference can be used in various ways to provoke a reaction in the analyst, which then confirms the patient's primitive experience of the object relationship. In fact, he would like to change the analyst's formal role. In that case, it is no longer a matter of communication or dialogue; it is a power struggle. Due to the onset of projective and introjective phenomena, communication becomes complex, like a house of mirrors, and the analyst runs the risk of identifying with the patient's internal objects.

The interpretations provided in a later stage of therapy may be strongly challenged and rejected because they change the fixed framework of the patient's own image and are experienced as being persecutory. The destructive narcissism goes so far as to block any channel of communication.

Another difficulty may be the lack of continuity in emotional contact (fluctuations in the transference) as well as the alternation between the sense of being and non-being. The issues highlighted in dreams or in the previous session are abandoned and sometimes not acknowledged as their own. Thus, any hope of making progress is abandoned and the patient finds himself, once again, cut off from life.

In the transference of my patient Sara, there were attempts to seek closeness and understanding as an expression of her infantile needy parts, but these were quickly replaced by the need to establish herself as an adult, as a grandiose subject to be admired, also able to reject the other.

Due to these fluctuations, it was difficult to perceive the continuity of the relationship in the countertransference, or to understand the truth or the coherence of the verbal messages. So the countertransference changed, from acknowledging a genuine need for contact, represented by an assiduous effort to stay in the analytical relationship, all the way to feelings of being paralyzed in a meaningless situation, devoid of any possible development.

In cases of autism, the need for more frequent sessions is often questioned, but the pace of the sessions, with as few breaks as possible between one and the other, should help the patient bear the separation and the fear of loss that is linked to death, and at the same time, to preserve the hope that new contact may be possible. The thread of the relational bond is thus maintained, reinforcing memory and attention to the emerging feelings. The patient's concrete interpretation of reality and use of projective identification will lead her to think that the reason for more frequent sessions lies in the analyst's financial needs.

Another way the analyst may be provoked in the transference is by being treated like an autistic object or an appendage, which prevents the acknowledgement of separation. The patient provides material that does not give rise to interpretation; he/she does not make associations; he/she organizes everything in a repetitive, sometimes obsessive way so as to control the other's feelings and spark anger. Or, by becoming himself/herself an autistic object, with repetitive and meaningless behaviour, he/she engages the object so that it remains attached, feels boredom, and thus destroys the fertility of thought. He or she doesn't miss a chance to prove that he/she has not benefited from the analytical work, but has actually become doubtful and depressed.

The transference may also take place outside the analytic space, in other contexts, such as through relationships that are repeatedly described during the sessions, or in the body. The lack of interpersonal communication, in times of strong resistance, can actually transfer the negative transference to the body, for example, by creating a dividing wall (with gastric pain, vertigo, headaches and vomiting, psychosomatic illnesses or skin eczema). In this case, the resistance to the analyst is evaded by innumerable and repeated diagnostic examinations to prove the presence of organic malfunctions responsible for the symptoms.

The transference can also be projected into the analyst's body, causing discomfort, functional disorders, numbness or sleep during the sessions.

Common to these patients are irregular moods and affective states when relating to others, all due to unprocessed meanings.

10.2 The analyst faced with the emptiness of autistic states

In therapy with adults, as opposed to therapy with children, the autistic experiences of moments of crisis can actually be described, since language is more developed. This can inform us about the mental states evoked by the unconscious. But in any case, the difficulty in establishing a relationship of emotional closeness makes contact particularly evasive.

In the acute phase, the patient feels alone within a body devoid of physical strength or mental resources, lost in an unknown world. He presents an image of great weakness and inability to think. The analytical relationship seems to turn into a state of helplessness and human suffering, with no possibility of development. The adult patient is like a helpless and suffering infant: there is no internal supporting object to communicate with. The relationship with the therapist is without any real emotional contact. In this way, anxieties that come from normal human communication are avoided. The most frequent terms used are: emptiness, fear of falling in an endless space, feeling of being made of air, without any strength. The analyst wonders how to restore corporeal boundaries that can keep the patient's body and mind together.

Furthermore, the analyst has to go to great lengths to withstand the feelings of desolation and emptiness and not be overwhelmed by the mental death projected on him. He must instead try to transmit vitality and serenity. No easy task.

In this acute situation of suffering, one wonders how to offer help in the realm of analytic therapy. Alvarez (1992) states that, in this experience, one feels the urgency to offer emergency care for the patient's extreme desperation.

In the encounter with varying degrees of disintegration, the analyst's internal state is put to the test because of the variability of the emerging mental states at various moments. When the patient experiences a state of disintegration, he presents a condition of psychic emptiness and desolation. This total sense of painful loneliness is sometimes not attributed by the patient to specific external events, and there seems to be nothing that can mitigate this. The state of deep crisis leads us into a timeless atmosphere, with no solution, no feelings of attachment, no passion or love, often in a state of boredom.

Khan (1964) sees this type of boredom as an attempt to petrify time in which there are no hopes that something might happen, only catastrophic fears. Boredom might result from a dissociation between emotions and cognition. It may arise from personal events that have not been symbolized, and it is hard to identify a comprehensible connection with the emotions experienced by the patient.

Bergstein (2009) differentiates the analyst's dreamy state and evenly suspended attention from a particular state of discomfort felt with autistic patients that arises from meaningless silence and extreme intellectual idleness. The analyst inwardly suffers from boredom and emptiness, as I have already indicated.

This author suggests that boredom can signal the presence of encapsulated parts in which the two-dimensional primitive experiences that prevail could not be processed because of primitive environmental difficulties. The adhesive identification has not permitted an experience of separation and of being two, and the analyst's boredom can be experienced as the re-enactment of a primitive experience of emptiness and lack of an object relationship.

So the analyst is confronted with her or his own deepest feelings, associated with her/his archaic experience of emptiness or loneliness, and looks within the Self for those emotional elements that might be called to mind in order to restore an internal climate of strength and well-being.

The patient does not transmit thoughts or fantasies, but tries to make the analyst feel what he himself feels through projective identification. He repeats through transference those primitive emotions that belong to a pre-verbal – or, in any case, very early – period, in which he did not ask for verbal responses from the mother, but instead asked for gestures to help him come out of his distress. At that time of his life, it was the mother who served as a device to hear and think. In this situation, the analyst must refrain from doing, as would happen in the actual maternal situation, but instead has to undertake greater mental and emotional work by attempting to understand the profound infantile situation present in the session.

If it is the case in the real situation of the session, we will try to provide the patient with our presence, closeness and emotional attention, watching every bodily or verbal message given by the patient. We will use our imagination to translate this into psychic meanings and thus create, as it were, a loom on which to weave the analytical process. This means offering (or temporarily loaning) our own fantasies or thoughts, paying attention to the slightest detail.

The transference, in these moments of crisis, recreates a deadly trauma and brings up a message that cannot be processed at the level of verbal communication. At that moment the transference is negative because its roots lie in this deadly situation, linked to the body, the patient having experienced in the early days of life the lack of satisfactory responses from the surrounding environment.

With autistic subjects whose mental life has not developed in a symbolic sense, Bion (the mother's alpha function, 1962) suggests that therapists should use their imagination and fill in the alpha function rather than offer interpretations, because the symbolic process is not yet in place. The work is to fill with meaning what was previously lacking in meaning until the patient is able to attribute meanings of her/his own.

The recurring themes of boredom, internal death and emptiness which I have already mentioned stimulate the analyst to restore vitality with her/his own feelings, but she/he must be aware that if this activity is too intense or too prolonged, it will make the patient too passive.

Moving from a phase of absolute desperation to a more evolved one, the patient takes possession of the answers given by the analyst that he experiences as clarifying (or later as interpretations) and uses them as if they were his own, only then to eliminate them in moments of anger. For her/him everything is her/his rightful due, she/he does not feel gratitude, as in the primitive early experiences with the mother: this cannibalistic tendency holds sway. This means one must as an analyst find a balance between helping the suffering parts and providing an activating stimulus, while simultaneously considering the optimal moment for intervention.

Alvarez (1992) says that autistic children who have lost not just hope but also parts of the Ego have a need to be 'reclaimed'. It is important to understand why they are spurred into being boring and adhesive, rather than continuing as an analyst to be an autistic object with no vital abilities.

Alvarez (2012) highlights the need to differentiate between children who have had primitive experiences with an undifferentiated, dead, absent or obtuse object, from patients who withdraw defensively from the relationship. Depending on the case, one will have to use different techniques: either activate a potential capacity for mental life or facilitate integration with interpretative activity. This also applies to adults.

In these situations, taking the place of the patient's thinking means helping them internalize the way they seek their own meanings, and not giving them our own meanings as a model to be copied. We do not know if what we say makes sense for the patient or not. The important thing is that the analyst wanders freely with her/his imagination, moving away from boredom towards creativity. In this way the patient can glimpse, through the other, that it is possible to grow and have an internal dialogue.

10.3 The ups and downs of countertransference

We have found that, in the therapies of patients with autistic residues, it takes a long time to dismantle defensive barriers first erected in childhood. As the sessions proceed and the analytical work moves forward, primitive manoeuvres come back into play, obstructing alliances and communication. These difficulties vary depending on the different levels of the patient's mental state and habitual defensive constructions.

Regarding therapy with children with autism, Alvarez (1992, 2012) notes the technical implications that arise from the huge variability of countertransference experiences induced by the type of defences put in place by the patient. The type of intervention needs to change each time. I have found that these observations made by Alvarez about children with autism are also true when working with autism in adults; nonetheless, it is important to consider the different level of personality development and the means of expression used.

In countertransference, the 'facts' may be confusing and the experiences produce physical and psychological pain.

For the analyst, the initial confusion in the first sessions arises from an apparent normality and adequate adaptation to reality, which masks the hidden autistic parts.

Further on, when things start to progress, the analyst may be confused by the fact that she does not perceive a link between the fragile, needy part and the one that is acted out, which may be provocative or violent. This determines – in the countertransference – opposite and unexplainable feelings. At times, when the vindictive part, full of hate, prevails in the countertransference, the analyst starts to doubt the patient's suffering part, which she had perceived before.

Another confusing element is the lack of modesty and tact in the initial phases of the encounter. If, on the one hand, it is possible to perceive the difficulty of emotional contact in the immediate relationship, on the other hand these shortcomings seem incongruent. They express the lack of regulation of the emotional distance between one and the other.

The Italian word *pudore*[1] has a relational meaning because it refers to a way of relating to one another. Apart from its significance in the context of sexuality, it contains a symbolic meaning (Selz, 2003). Pudore is usually a feeling assigned to the exhibition of the body, but here it refers to a problem regarding language as a means of presenting oneself.

I believe that lack of pudore can be seen as an excessive ease in talking about intimate memories before the analytical relationship has developed, as a display of the nudity of one's internal emotional world. It does not convey complete confidence in the other, rather it indicates the absence of an interior space with borders and meanings that usually characterizes reservation. Unlike the word shame, which expresses a narcissistic element, pudore is connected to object relationships, personal differentiation and the measurement of optimal distance, depending on the situation and the roles.

Similarly, we may find a lack of tact, which represents the lack of any immediate intuition of the complex meanings and nuances that come into play in the language directed towards the other. This, too, may be linked to a disorder in symbolization, in the sense of the true meaning or the opportunity to use an offensive phrase. Evidence of this is the fact that, as the analysis progresses and the process of symbolization starts to be applied, the patient is able to point out, for example, an emotional nuance grasped in the analyst's language. After years, for example, one patient could remember and confess to having really heard the sweetness of a word the analyst had spoken, which had the effect of being a charitable gift.

A difficult obstacle to the development of analytical thinking is obsessive ideation, in which the fixed nature of the symptoms can signify an ancient attempt to overcome the fear of fragmentation. However, at the same time, it prevents the process of separation, which is essential for individuation and symbolization. The acceptance of separation as a space between the Self and the other rekindles the fear of falling into an empty space. The despair of the past is re-experienced, until a protective, safe and stable object has been introjected. The difficulty also lies in the need to renounce the idea of an ideal, total and unattainable emotional relationship, in the service of dealing with a real bond and the emergence of depressive phase. The dilemma inherent in obsessive thinking also creates difficulties in ending the analysis, when real separation must be faced.

When the defences created in order to avoid primitive anxieties and despair are accompanied by various forms of addiction, the relationship with the analyst is hugely hampered by the evasion, through acting-out, occurring outside the sessions. The need to act concretely is due to the need to demonstrate one's power; furthermore, the development of addictions substitutes the need for human bonds. The consumption of drugs, smoke, food, alcohol and sex is an attempt to construct a source of well-being in lieu of affective relationships, and to control these as one wishes.

The continuous display, through the patient's speech, of the activities in the various areas of addiction is a way to provoke the analyst, making her/him a curious and powerless spectator. This sparks anger in the analyst regarding the abuse, the sadistic feelings evoked, and the subsequent desire to get rid of the patient. It is important to defend the need for personal well-being and continue to process the countertransference.

When talking of patients with autism and their skilful defensive manoeuvres, Tustin (1986) suggests the need for the therapist to be firm in her/his role, and possibly stop the use of autistic modalities, while remaining empathic with the hidden suffering parts. In her view, the analytical relationship must have a guide, in the sense of a benevolent paternal authority. Patients often attempt to defeat the analyst, as if they were in combat against an enemy.

These patients fight the sadness and despair of primitive experiences with the reactions of mania and omnipotence that have characterized all their activities and interpersonal relationships. If the analyst mentions these modes as an ancient way of psychic survival, the patient considers her or him to be a killjoy, and becomes all the more convinced of the goodness of this excitement. She or he claims it as her or his expression of vitality, youth and good health, and projects onto the analyst her or his depression, thus denying it. The persistent links between these different forms of defence are interwoven and mutually reinforced. Without constant excitement, life loses its value. Similarly, the use of a continuous erection over time is enhanced and confused with the ability to love and with the continuity of feelings of love.

Finally, when psychopathic characteristics prevail, or in other words, when the hate, the need for revenge and violence prevail in the internal world, it becomes difficult for the analyst to keep in mind the hypothesis that there may be a part made up of good feelings, beyond the aggressiveness perceived. Docker-Drysdale (1990), cited by Alvarez, notes that in cases of an early lack of love and containment, the existence of love cannot be known.

The hatred of the psychotic part attacks the bond and displays hatred for feelings and connections with thought. Hatred is seen only in others, but it cannot be acknowledged within oneself. Thus the analyst starts to be considered dangerous, as the patient becomes aware of her/his own truth. The attack on the analyst and on her/his ability to think may be open and violent, or masked with skilful manipulation and seduction, and in any case it is always aimed at destroying the real bond. This behaviour is supported by omnipotence and the narcissistic need to win over the other as well as the need for concrete revenge.

Symington (2007) describes the dangers of the feelings of countertransference when faced with the behaviour of psychopathic patients. The analyst may respond with collusion, disbelief, denial and condemnation with regards to the feelings evoked by the patient. Alvarez adds the fear that some patients evoke in their therapist. Only by accepting and processing these feelings can the relationship progress. The patient is excited by the fact he can evoke these feelings in the analyst, and takes on a challenge to maintain this course of the relationship.

Considering that these are adults who have a certain degree of relational ability in their daily social lives, I have experienced that it is important to face one's fear of being defeated on a human and professional level. Through their contempt and attempt to destroy our thinking ability, these patients evoke disturbances in our professional identity. It is important to move forward in the analytical relationship with courage, rather than piety or false availability. This means not forgetting the fragility of the abused part, but also not lending oneself to being continuously abused. It is important to respond to the patient's well-rooted manipulative ability with the power of the truth of our feelings, which have been acknowledged and processed, without evading the possibility of the failure of analysis.

10.4 McDougall and Green: about countertransference

During supervision sessions with Joyce McDougall, I was able to discuss my countertransferential experiences in my work with adult patients who had autistic residues, which felt very close to her experience with neurotic, borderline and psychosomatic patients who had asked her for long analyses.

McDougall (1978, 1982, 1989) named them 'désaffectés' because, in her opinion, as a consequence of primitive suffering, they separated early on from their feelings. McDougall claims that they reduced all emotional investment in their lives and built strong defences against 'feelings', including through somatization. She says that their transference is always negative and determines countertransference responses characterized by confusion, anxiety, boredom and other disturbing emotions. McDougall suggests that, when these patients were children, they had to take refuge in a deadly world in order to survive, and this is reproduced in the transference.

In times of great distress and difficulty in the course of analysis with these patients, McDougall analyses the progression of her countertransference, and questions analysts' motivations in taking on this type of patient and the motivation of the very analysands in undertaking analysis. In fact, these patients seem to ask for help, but in the transference they behave in such a way as to make the other person powerless to help, trying to prove that they are stronger than the analyst and that they know how to destroy her/him. It seems that in the transference they try to establish an archaic bond that does not foresee separation, and so they try to cancel any differences with the analyst because they wish to be completely fused with her/him. However, such fusion would be equally deadly, devoid of creativity and any exchange of symbolic thought. The anxiety, emotions and confusion are difficult for the analyst to bear, and as I have said may lead to boredom. Hence, in the countertransference, the analyst experiences the twofold message of pain and confusion received by the child, which prompted her/him to reduce his vitality.

McDougall (1989) suggests that:

> it takes patience (Winnicott-style holding – he talked of 'waiting and waiting' in The Use of the Object), and this implies the need not only to wait and dominate 'our malevolent neutrality', but also to retain the other, if necessary; in other words, to maintain the analytical framework intact (to the extent that this can allow the analytical process to move forward). Thus, we have to be able to contain and process our emotional relationships in the hope that the other comes to believe that she/he will be given sufficient time and space, so that a thought might be born: a thought other than that of an angry need for revenge or the expectation of total reparation. This task poses particular risks, as we are confronted with a dimension of internal death that infiltrates the analytic discourse and threatens our vitality.

Similarly, regarding the difficulties encountered by the analyst in the countertransference, and its importance in therapeutic interventions, Green (1986) describes the 'dead mother complex' to indicate the child's experience following the stripping of experience offered by a depressed mother (caused by a more or less symbolic bereavement). This leads to the development of a latent depression, unacknowledged as a conflict. The child goes from a known and already experienced condition of love and the feeling of being loved, to the perception of a cold and insensitive nucleus.

Green warns that, in these cases, one should neither intervene prematurely by repeating the intrusion of a bad object, nor abstain from intervening, because that would replicate the inaccessibility of the good object. It is better to keep an open space in which the patient can experience things without meaning, alongside things with many meanings: a position of investigation and enquiry should be highlighted. This would bring out two aspects of the mind: one in which there are many meanings, and another in which there is a fluctuating state with no meanings, with neurotic and psychotic parts, with interpretations, or an abstention from defences. The idea is to find a way to move beyond the experience of emotional death, to create vitality in a realm of previous emptiness and desolation, and facilitate the attainment of hidden potential.

From McDougall's and Green's experiences, we can infer that these patients, who appear 'super-normal', place the analyst in a situation of exclusion and reject the analyst's efforts to think about them. Simultaneously, they require a fusional regression and ask the analyst to do the thinking for them.

Reed *et al.* (2013, p. 12) summarize the characteristics of Green's thought (1975, p. 6) in three points:

> 1st – There exists 'a confusion between subject and object, with a blurring of the limits of the self'.
> 2nd – 'The particular mode of symbolization is derived from a dual organization of patient and analyst.'
> 3rd – 'There is a need for structural integration through the object.'

Note

1 Translator's note: the closest English translations are: modesty, discretion or decency. In French, it is *pudeur*.

References

Alvarez, A. (1992) *Live company*, London and New York: Tavistock and Routledge.
Alvarez, A. (2012) *The thinking heart*, London and New York: Routledge.
Bergstein, A. (2009) 'On boredom: a close encounter with encapsulated parts of the psyche', *International Journal Psychoanalysis*, 90, 613–631.
Bion, W. R. (1962) 'A theory of thinking'. In *Second thoughts: selected papers of psychoanalysis* (pp. 110–199), New York: Jason Aronson, 1967.

Docker-Drysdale, B. (1990) *The provision of primary experience: Winnicottian work with children and adolescents*, London: Free Association Books.

Green, A. (1975) 'The analyst, symbolization and absence in the analytic setting: on changes in analytic practises and experience. In memory of D. W. Winnicott', *International Journal of Psychoanalysis*, 56, 1–22.

Green, A. (1986) 'The dead mother'. In *On private madness* (pp. 142–173), London: Hogarth.

Isaacs, S. (1952) 'The nature and function of phantasy'. In J. Riviere (ed.), *Developments in psycho-analysis* (pp. 67–121), London: Hogarth.

Khan, M. (1964) 'Ego distortion, cumulative trauma, and the role of reconstruction in the analytic situation', *International Journal of Psychoanalysis*, 45, 272–279.

McDougall, J. (1978) *Plea for a measure of abnormality*, New York: International Universities Press.

McDougall, J. (1982) 'Alexithymia, psychosomatosis and psychosis', *International Journal of Psychoanalysis and Psychotherapy*, 9, 379–388.

McDougall, J. (1989) 'One body for two'. In *Theaters of the body* (pp. 140–161), London: Free Association Books.

Reed, G. S., Levine, H. B. and Scarfone, D. (2013) 'Introduction: from a universe of presences to a universe of absences'. In H. B. Levine, G. S. Reed and D. Scarfone (eds), *Unrepresented states and the construction of meaning: clinical and theoretical* (pp. 3–17), London: Karnac.

Selz, M. (2003) *La pudeur, un lieu de liberté*, Paris: Buchet Chastel.

Symington, N. (2007) *Becoming a person*, London: Karnac.

Tustin, F. (1986) *Autistic barriers in neurotic patients*, London: Karnac.

Chapter 11

The challenges of working with autistic traits

> If I have made any discovery of value, it is due more to patient attention than to any other talent. Genius is patience.
>
> (Isaac Newton, 1642–1727)

11.1 Patience as a working tool and the need for self-analysis

I had the opportunity to encounter the concept of 'being patient' early on in my childhood: my family lived during the time of a political regime, in which one could not freely express thoughts that were different from those imposed, nor carry out one's own social and personal ideals. I could see in the adults close to me – family members and their friends – that the patient wait for change prevailed over action. At that time, patience seemed to me to be linked more to the idea of repression or resignation or fear of persecution. Later on, I realized that patience was associated with tolerating frustration and contained high potential: through patience one could develop the ability to adapt to reality and the tenacity to preserve it with an eventual outcome in mind. I understood that because of the external social situation, one had to wait and think about how to strengthen the hope for change and how to conduct one's life without renouncing intellectual freedom. Patience, combined with prudence, and the study of issues with ongoing reflection, was for that generation a non-violent weapon that permitted them to resist the dictatorship, preserve their ideals and survive in difficult times. (It is said that one needs to arm oneself with patience when embarking on a difficult task.)

In that case, the waiting time was not empty; it was full of efforts to understand, to study and to foster bonds of solidarity and friendship with people who shared the same ideals. This enabled people to process thoughts and projects, while paying close attention to the development of events. Years later, during my adolescence at the end of the regime, I could see that the patient wait, united with hope, had formed the basis for a process of change in the political situation and the achievement of desired projects over time.

Patience may be difficult to accept in youth, because one learns patience over time and through personal experience. Eventually, it comes to be considered indispensable in the maturing of internal projects, without the individual being overcome by the youthful urge to hurry, to understand everything at once, to act impulsively and to establish the Self in a way which may be premature. The concept of patience is connected to that of waiting, and therefore to the concept of time.

Patience is developed with tranquillity, peace and tolerance, and it also accompanies humility in the ability to recognize one's limits and admit that one cannot know everything (Trevi, 2008).

In the realm of analytical thinking, Bion (1970, 1973) talks about 'negative capability' (a phrase first coined by the British poet Keats) and he introduces the term patience to refer to the analyst's empathic ability to wait and tolerate frustration.

Lacan suggests that in training analysis the analyst learns to 'touch and know the field and the feeling of being absolutely lost, a level in which anxiety is a protection in itself' (1994, p. 381).

Confusion arises when one realizes that in the analytical couple one is alone in the effort of finding a way to communicate constructively. In extreme cases, the analyst has to detach him or herself from theoretical knowledge, reconsider his or her subjectivity and continue self-analysis to find a possible way to communicate with the patient.

Ferenczi (1930–1932, p. 218) believes that self-analysis can be completed only with the patient's help. By going back through one's history, one will retrace feelings and events, some of which have already been analysed and some of which have not; this creates a waiting time which is needed to process all these elements. The work of self-analysis leads one to break away from the senses, from the perceivable presence of the object, and to represent these through language and memory. In analytical work with patients that reach deep levels of disintegration, the analyst has to retrace the path of his or her own subjectivity to find the right approach. This requires a revision of what they have already analysed, but is also confronted with problematic parts of the Self that have not yet been analysed.

When one is met with strong resistance and continuous contrasting points of view with the patient, or when there is a threat that the relationship will be interrupted, the idea of the analyst's failure – and that of the patient – comes into play. Winnicott (1971, 1989) proposes a paradox, namely that 'a successful analysis must include a delirium of failure and a patient's reaction to analysis as a failure'. He believes that in this case the analyst must accept that not everything about himself has been analysed and that he has no theoretical or absolute truths. Thus, the analyst's subjectivity is at stake. When speaking of the 'unthought known', Bollas (1989) refers to the un-analysed remains in the analyst.

For example, severe difficulties in the relationship create fantasies of termination and internal representations of how the patient should react to certain events or interpretations. In these situations, the analysis of one's own narcissism becomes essential in order to cope with the continuing threat of failure.

During analytical work with mental states of a contiguous-autistic or paranoid-schizoid nature, waiting patiently allows the analyst to gather elements which have emerged from the various levels of the patient's personality, and keep them suspended before order can be made out of the chaos of the material. To these elements, one must add one's own thoughts or unresolved questions.

This state of waiting allows one to find the most appropriate way to intervene. Waiting patiently is not a passive or empty experience; it is a lively phase in which, alongside differences of opinion and misunderstandings, one can find personal questions, always supported by the basic faith in psychoanalysis as a path towards knowledge. Patience in psychotherapy provides a space and a time to retrieve buried archaic emotions. The analyst's patience helps him or her to endure the patient's attacks and the long wait needed to reach an understanding; it also helps the patient to maintain a consistent inner picture of the ongoing work.

One might notice that in an effort to strengthen their individuality, and alongside their emotional suffering, these patients have increased their knowledge from books, from the internet or by copying social models, and this has provoked pride, presumption and unfounded narcissism. In this way, they have tried to avoid interpersonal relationships as a means of developing their subjectivity. Thus, they see patience as a sign of weakness or as the inability to act.

11.2 Main difficulties

Unlike children with autism or others forms of psychological damage, adults with autistic nuclei are able to lead seemingly normal social lives and speak correctly and fluently. This might lead the analyst to adopt an interpretive approach regarding a patient's resistance. But such an approach would be premature, and is not indicated in these cases.

Many authors have described the persistence of repetitive autistic manoeuvres used to avoid depression or the shame of the depressive phase. The protective armour can be represented in various ways, including persistent anxiety that makes progress impossible, or psychosomatic disorders that nullify the mental development process, or even the easy external turn to addiction (McDougall, 1989, 1972). In some cases, the analytic couple is turned into an immobile autistic object that the patient utilizes to demonstrate an ability to form an affective alliance while, at the same time, seeking to underline the impossibility of good therapeutic results. (Klein, 1980; Tustin, 1984, 1986, 1990; Innes-Smith, 1987; Odgen, 1989; Gomberoff et al., 1990; Mitrani, 1996).

Such patients can also express a lack of symbolization, and may not see the analytic relationship as being affectively significant. They can, in addition, possess deficits in time-space concepts, as well as difficulties with body image, distance and proximity. As regards verbal communication, topics may be monotonous, mainly alluding to concrete facts and reality, with the accompanying denial of any possibility of mental work.

This evident lack may initially relate to the lack of understanding and acceptance of the rules of the setting. Some patients arrive with delays of up to half an hour, thus reducing the time of work and controlling the waiting analyst. The same holds true for the payment of the sessions.

With neurotic patients we might interpret these delays as a devaluation of the analyst, a denial of dependence, excitement due to the omnipotent control of the analyst, and aggression in the transference, etc. However, in these cases, this particular type of interpretation would be premature, and certainly useless. None of the attempts to find some meaning in this repetitive behaviour is effective. I subsequently realized that the concept of time was not experienced in the usual sense of an internal coordinate of one's being. The emotional and social significance of the encounter simply did not exist in such patients.

In the case of late arrivals, we can see the attempt to deny the presence of the other in the therapeutic couple and narcissistically occupy the whole relational field.

In these cases, containment can be difficult, because the patient's behaviour interferes with the progress of the analytic work and its essential rules. Emphasizing the rules may inflame a desire to rebel, as this reawakens the subject of infantile dependence and hatred towards internal objects.

Sara attempted to manipulate the situation by telling me that late arrivals allowed her to enjoy a moment of relaxation. This demonstrates the process of projective identification and, moreover, it shows a transformation of the truth of the encounter.

As the analysis progresses and the affective relationship is strengthened, such patients themselves become punctual and recognize their previous lack of consideration, and their tendency to disregard the analyst in a justification for their previous delays.

In terms of the concept of the relationship in itself, the link with the other is only possible in their actual presence. If the analyst moves away physically, the patient cannot hold inside the representation and the meaning of the encounter.

The idea of absence cannot be tolerated, because separation is experienced as the final disappearance of the other, or the patient's own death. Separation for the weekend or for holidays is not well tolerated and may be followed by acting-out.

Patients with addiction to drugs, alcohol, sex and gambling easily flee from the analytic field, with frequent acting-out. These kinds of behaviour are difficult to eliminate since, in the past, they represented an escape from the thinking Self and a safe haven, in the manner of autistic objects. Tustin (1986, 1988, 1990) noted the presence of autistic nuclei in neurotic behaviour, or in patients with addiction to drugs and sex. She pointed out that the perverse mechanisms in autism are very resistant to treatment. Indeed, in these patients, bodily and tactile sensations have a defensive function employed in order to avoid a vacuum.

These sensations may offer a sense of being, but they also result in chronic psychosomatic disorders.

Particularly, in the case of sex addiction, the continuous search for sex results from the idea of not being able to survive without these types of sensations, which provide a feeling of power and self-confidence. (See Chapter 5: Sara) The absence of self-worth is masked by behaviour that stands for 'personal success' in today's society and is an affirmation of one's value, mirrored by messages given in today's consumer society. The inability to attribute feelings of love to any interpersonal relationship that are ideally interminable in time is associated with the need for concrete things. Relinquishing the repetition of this behaviour triggers the fear of disappearing and losing one's identity: repetitive actions express the obsessive defences of autism. Success in affective relationships is attributed to the actual number of partners, which replaces the sense of enrichment, which can be experienced between the couple. This, however, gives rise to a fragmentation of relational experiences, and promotes once again the experience of a vacuum, an experience that does not contain depressive feelings for the object. Any discussion about the meaning of addiction is interpreted by such patients as a prohibition or a moral imperative. The analyst is considered to be a puritan or a killjoy and is therefore disputed and then eliminated from the patient's mind.

In terms of the difficulties that arise, I would like to point out the need to differentiate between patients with unconscious autistic nuclei and those of a schizoid type, in whom the nucleus of primitive autistic experience has been recognized by the patient and even transformed into a permanent pillar of the personality.

One could say that what develops is a form of addiction to these negative experiences, contributing to the creation of one's own 'bad' internal objects. In this case, analytic work can be long and difficult because of the anaesthetizing effect the patient uses in affective experience as a primitive defence. I might call this 'addiction' to bad affective experiences (internal objects) because, in spite of any attempt to think through the concept of a past time, the new, living and analytical experiences of the present and the whole tone and mood of the relationship cannot change (Steiner, 1993).

Fairbairn (1956) points out that, for the child, bad internal objects are better than no objects at all: given the degree of his dependence and needs, he cannot relinquish them. The patient transforms this experience of rejection and absence of love into one representative part of his own identity that cannot be relinquished. He therefore transforms himself into a rigid figure, disillusioned with the external world, with persistent feelings of scarcity, always ashamed to ask for help and demonstrating pervasive hostility. Indeed, he wastes his life reproducing the characteristics of these unsatisfactory internal objects in his behaviour towards himself and others.

The way these patients live becomes an interminable form of seeking a way of infantile revenge. The analysis is sought out as a form of help, since the analytic relationship represents a couple kept together by the patient's will. Indeed, the principle aim is to exercise the right to express one's own anger and dissatisfaction and to paralyze the persecutory other.

It can therefore take a long time for analytic work to bring about a change from the patient's position of victim to one where an active role in the present can shape a new self-image, and interpersonal relationships may be experienced in a different way.

References

Bion, B. W. (1970) *Attention and interpretation*, London: Tavistock Publications.
Bion, B. W. (1973) *Brazilian lectures, 1*, Rio de Janeiro: Imago Editora.
Bollas, C. (1989) *The shadow of the object*, New York: Columbia University Press.
Fairbairn, W. R. D. (1956) 'Re-evaluating some basic concepts'. In D. Scharff and E. F. Birtles (eds), *From instinct to self: selected papers of W.E.D. Farbairn, vol. 1: clinical and theoretical papers* (pp. 129–138), London: Jason Aronson, 1994.
Ferenczi, S. (1930–1932) 'Notes and fragments'. In *Final contribution to the problems and methods of psychoanalysis* (pp. 219–279), London: Hogarth, 1955.
Gomberoff, M. J., Noemi, C. C. and Pualuan de Gomberoff, L. (1990) 'The autistic object: its relationship with narcissism in the transference and countertransference of neurotic and borderline patients', *International Journal of Psychoanalysis*, 71, 249–259.
Innes-Smith, J. (1987) 'Pre-oedipal identification and the cathexis of autistic objects in the aetiology of adult psychopathology', *International Journal of Psychoanalysis*, 68, 405–414.
Klein, S. (1980) 'Autistic phenomena in neurotic patients', *International Journal of Psychoanalysis*, 61, 395–401.
Lacan, J. (1994) *The four fundamental concepts of psycho-analysis*, London and New York: State University of New York Press.
McDougall, J. (1972) 'Création et déviations sexuelle', *Revue française de psychoanalyse*, 4.
McDougall, J. (1989) 'One body for two'. In *Theaters of the body* (pp. 140–161), London: Free Association Books.
Mitrani, J. (1996) *A framework of the Imaginary*, London: Karnac.
Ogden, T. H. (1989) *The primitive edge of experience*, London: Karnac.
Steiner, J. (1993) *Psychic retreats*, London: Routledge.
Trevi, M. (2008) *Dialogo sull'arte del dialogo*, Milano: Feltrinelli.
Tustin, F. (1984) 'Autistic shapes', *International Journal of Psychoanalysis*, 11(3), 279–290.
Tustin, F. (1986) *Autistic barriers in neurotic patients*, London: Karnac.
Tustin, F. (1988) '"To be or not to be" – a study of autism', *Winnicott Studies*, 3, 43–55.
Tustin, F. (1990) *The protective shell in children and adults*, London: Karnac.
Winnicott, D. W. (1971) *Playing and reality*, London: Tavistock Publications.
Winnicott, D. W. (1989) *On human nature*, London: Routledge.

Chapter 12

Suggestions for therapeutic interventions

12.1 Ways of intervening

First: the vitalizing level

I use the same approach in the intervention that Alvarez (2012) describes in treatment with children and adolescents with various types of autism, because I was able to spontaneously experiment a trajectory of these steps with adult patients, and therefore take in Alvarez's suggestions.

Alvarez defines the vitalizing level of work as being one used with very damaged children in whom both the Self and the internal objects have been damaged.

This level of work precedes descriptive and explanatory levels, and is related to situations such as autism, dissociation, despairing apathy and emptiness of mind.

In adult patients with autistic nuclei, this kind of intervention will be suitable during the crisis of disintegration.

The patient's failure to be 'in tune' to thoughts and feelings should lead us to question his or her ability to listen before we intervene. We must first ponder how the patient's experience resonates in us so as to be able to make a contact with him and establish a relationship.

The internal objects might be uninteresting, undervalued, useless, mindless, perversely excitable, or even dead. The main function of the analyst is to provide first aid, offering closeness, transmitting vitality and awakening a thinking function in the more passive and despairing patient. In these cases, Alvarez (1980, 1992) suggests an act of reclamation by the therapist in response to a powerful feeling of urgency. Alvarez's concept of 'reclamation' can be useful in cases where the atrophy of internal objects prevails and the patient must be called back to life. We should not forget that these patients are often identified with dead objects. (See Irene's case in Chapter 6.)

Our involvement, owing to the intensity of the anxiety about fragmentation and death, should be manifested by an alert and active proximity to the patient, who then perceives our interest in them. Both bodily behaviour and verbal communication can provide some hint to stimulate a dialogue.

The analyst sets in motion the sense of a close and active presence, a tone of voice that expresses strength and certainty and vigilant attention to the patient's reactions. She also has to discourage the patient's passivity and the tendency to be addicted to repetitive behaviour. The analyst's personality and her mental state testify to her vitality, and her subjectivity comes into play.

In the cases of Sara and Irene, my interventions were initially sparse, reduced to the indispensable, in order to make room for reflection. I felt it was important to detect any small and apparently insignificant detail in order to convey my attention and reinforce the fact that we were two people rather than one merged person. The continuity of the analyst's interest in the patient is at this point the most important therapeutic aid. It is also important not to let the patient remain in silence for too long, because their mind tends to be empty.

With the adult patient who relives primitive experiences, I feel it is important to provide a comfortable meeting place, rather in the way that Bick (1968) suggests with children, in order to facilitate an integration of objects in the child.

The consulting room assumes importance as the patient's internal representation of the analyst and his space. One of my autistic patients at the beginning of our meetings would ask me to turn on the light, even when there was no need of it, in order to experience more warmth in our conversation. Was it the cold sensation of the previous separation that demanded more warmth? Was his internal coldness projected onto my room?

I used to use a perfume from an infuser, and she would complain about any absence or change in this. This made me think about the role of sensations in the process of infants' attachment, and the identification with the sensations of a familiar environment.

I also tried to avoid noises from the external environment and any interruptions of the sessions, because of the patients' hypersensitivity and tendency to feel neglected. The patient therefore will have the feeling that our focus is indeed on being together in the session.

Another important element is facilitating the integration of the sense of time, achieved by establishing regular sessions and a planned schedule. The apparent rigidity of the setting can represent a paternal aspect which helps establish limits (Houzel, 2001). However, since the schedules may frequently not be observed, despite reminders, the analyst has to wait until the patient arrives. In this situation, the containment function has to intervene and remain of upmost importance in the analyst's mind.

Containment aims to provide the patient with an experience of being accepted for a certain time, in contact, to enable him to begin to take on responsibility for himself and his own thoughts. The persistence in the analyst's mind of doubts and questions, impulses of despair or desires to give up provides the patient with an experience of a thinking model. Another human being is thinking about how to transform and fulfil the patient's needs in a more satisfactory way.

Paying specific attention to the changes in the patient, it is necessary to continuously observe our own moods, as well as the patient's verbal and non-verbal behaviour.

The way in which the body of the patient participates in the session is interesting. In the 'face to face' position, facial expressions will be helpful with respect to our interventions, and we can note the presence of stiffness or other bodily movements and positions. In terms of non-verbal behaviour, for example, the position or movement of the hands is particularly interesting. As I have previously mentioned, in the case of Sara, her hands were often used to accompany the words to express the shapes or measures of objects seen in her dreams as if words were not sufficient to express a concept.

When Sara listened to my interventions, which she would accept with great difficulty, she would rub her eyes incessantly with such violence that I imagined this expressed her violent feelings both against herself and against my words. In her case too, itching represented a bodily excitement that masked real feelings. But at this early level of work, it would not have been prudent of me to hint at her violence. After a long time, the same rubbing of her eyes became gentle and these movements seemed more like caresses and massages. It was thus possible to interpret the meaning of this behaviour (see Chapter 3).

These bodily behaviours can be interpreted only when we understand their meaning in order to help the integration of the body with the rest of the personality. But it is important to wait for the right timing, and not intervene too soon. At certain stages, it is also important to communicate the level of our own emotions in such a way that the experience of closeness and reciprocity of feeling is passed on to the patient, thus making him feel that he is heard and observed.

Another key element of containment is the analyst's voice, which signifies a bodily presence along with all other bodily signs. For example, variations in the tone of voice are important when speaking (funny, playful, calm, severe), and the spontaneous sounds that can express appreciation, understanding, sharing or wonder, as when we speak in a social situation. These communicative signs are important as fragments of an experience of affective contact; they can sometimes be points of convergence of feelings or thoughts, or at other times moments of disagreement. But they attest to the presence of the other's vitality and they then resonate in the patient's own Self. The analyst's language must also be simple and direct without the use of technical or intellectual words.

Patients are interested in the analyst's face and eyes: they are searching for his feelings or are projecting their own into him. Therefore, the verbal and non-verbal expressions are important in the short encounters at the beginning and end of the sessions, where mimicry and spontaneous communication of both parties is most evident.

For logistical reasons, my patient and I had to take a few steps in order to reach the exit from the consulting room, so we had a few minutes together. In the early stages of the analysis, at the end of a painful session, Sara's mood would veer towards mania, as if she could not possibly stay close to any feelings of depression or reflection. Sometimes she asked direct questions of a practical nature related to everyday problems that went way beyond the content of the sessions.

During the first periods of disintegration, at the time of separation, just before she left, I thought it was better to answer those questions simply, rather than give an immediate interpretation either then or in the next session, or be silent as would be the customary way. A classic analyst could have pointed out the patient's attempt to minimize leaving the setting, to devalue the analytic encounter, to turn it into a confidential conversation or to deny feelings of dependence. In order to reinforce Sara's fragile desire for a relationship, I thought instead of a simple answer, as an interpretation would have been inappropriate at that time. Moreover, if our purpose is to convey a new experience of how to establish a relationship – namely, of 'being together' – emphasizing the issue of non-compliance with the rules at that moment in time would not have made the process any easier. I did not think that frustration was appropriate at that moment, owing to her already confused state regarding her identity. In my opinion, her questions belonged to a functioning part of her personality, even though they were actually voiced just outside the analytical space. It seemed better not to interfere in her attempt to get closer to the analyst, and to accept her way of being. I also thought that, instead of an answer, an interpretation might have been dictated by my own narcissism, since I had been dethroned from the role of analyst. It was better not to put obstacles in the way when she was attempting the difficult task of accepting the analyst, and finding her own way of being with 'the other'.

Here we can see the difficulty in judging the right amount of interpersonal-affective distance, owing to Sara's lack of the ability to symbolize. It was only after a considerable time, in the few minutes spent together at the time of departure, that she could remain in the post-session atmosphere without trying to find a mirror image in me. She was beginning to contain within herself the impressions that emerged during the session and to accept her feelings regarding separation.

With respect to the classical rules, these modifications in the analyst's behaviour are determined by the patient's degree of disintegration. The flexibility of the analyst's behaviour depends on his or her emotional development, their personality and vitality, and especially the continuous analysis of their own narcissism. The confidence in the development of the analytic process is derived from theoretical knowledge, from learning in analytical schools and from keeping the containment of the rules of the setting in our mind.

I want to emphasize that the attitude of the analyst regarding the most disintegrated parts – namely, containment and first aid – should not be confused with an attitude of pity or passivity or a seductive proximity: these positions would on the contrary prevent us from pursuing our analytic search to identify defences.

These states of non-life or vacuum echo in the analyst's own mind as a return to primitive symbiotic fantasies. When the analyst is in touch with these parts of their inner world, they identify with the need for help and for maternal support in the first months of life. This then gives information about the necessity to take on the needs of the other. This approach and its necessary development draw attention to the concept of emotional closeness and attachment (Bowlby, 1979).

Second: the descriptive level

Emergence from the phase of disintegration will occur when the analyst has recognized and understood these primitive affective experiences. Gradually, the relationship with the analyst can be introjected by the patient.

When the phase of disintegration is over in which the emptiness and sense of loss of identity prevail, we may find ourselves faced with the patient's movement toward the more structured part of the personality, where different feelings such as arrogance, aggression, defiance or contempt prevail, according to the type of defence being used.

Nevertheless, the transition from a state of emptiness, loss of vitality and enormous dependence, to one of omnipotence and absolute superiority can occur rapidly, thus confusing the analyst. Once again, the analyst has to tolerate another situation of discomfort in his or her countertransference, due to the fact that they cannot immediately understand everything that is going on.

The scene of the analytic relationship changes and the analyst must find a way to intervene once again in a way that is different from the previous phases and from the classic analytical approach with adult patients.

Alvarez (2012) reflects on the therapeutic intervention after the phase of coming back to life, and proposes this descriptive level of intervention that aims to offer a wider range of meanings by clarifying some of the analyst's interpretations or the patient's words, offering one's own associations.

The patient's projections can be a useful means of communication for the analyst who, prior to this containment, can give the patient only part of the answers he is seeking. The rest will remain in the analyst's mind until the patient is able to understand and introject it. At this stage, it might be important to share with the patient some of his states of mind through empathic and amplified comments. Amplification will help introjection and develop the process of symbolization.

I would like to underline that, in approaching the communication of wealth of meanings that everyone can possess, one might encounter the resistance that the patient has built up over a lifetime, primarily the narcissism of autistic states. It poses as an obstacle in the acquisition of ideas that are different from one's own, as well as the ability to consider other points of views; it does not foster the ability to sustain stress from the surrounding world – in this case, from the analytical relationship. In reviewing their lifetime and coming up against other points of view, the patient will inevitably become aware of the mistakes they have made in evaluating past or present events. The fact that they were not able to recognize that they were projecting unconscious parts of themselves onto others is felt as an unacceptable frustration. Thus, we come to a state of permanent hostility towards the analyst and a situation of gridlock.

We can also suppose that, in this phase, the analyst's use of verbalization as a way to increase the range of meanings can be rejected by the patient because it is as a means of communication that is different from the patient's previous projective modality (Bion, 1958).

The analyst's skill lies in accepting the hostility towards change, and facilitating the possibility of introjecting new thoughts.

Transforming the interpersonal relationship, previously imagined simply as bodily proximity, requires the transformation of the concept of time and space from mechanical and pragmatic concepts to a mental space which is itself shaped by space and time. I have noticed in my work over many years that the deficit in symbolization mainly concerns the concepts of closeness and distance, space, time, and the internal and external body. The lack of symbolization manifests itself in the communication with subjects related solely to concreteness and reality.

In terms of the unfolding relationship, the link with the other is only possible when he is physically present. If the other moves away physically, it is impossible for the patient to keep in mind both the representation of the analyst and the affective significance of the previous meeting. Separation is felt as the final disappearance of the other and his own death.

These patients tend to think in terms of absolutes and opposites: omnipotence/impotence, good/bad, active/passive, able/unable. For example, one of the most difficult concepts to convey is that of the meaning of 'measurement', concerning both feelings as well as thoughts or actions. Behaviour is dependent on the specific situation as well as on one's habitual thoughts or feelings.

In the real world, one measures concrete objects based on conventional mathematical rules and comes up with a single, indisputable result. But when the word 'measurement' is used to refer to feelings or thoughts, and then to actions, there may be different interpretations, evaluations and judgements. Thus, the word 'measurement' contains the specificity of the subject that uses it. This leads to the notion of subjectivity and personal responsibility, which emerge from the experience of separation. This is an example of the difficulty in developing the process of symbolization.

We must not forget that autism involves immobility in interpersonal relationships and the tendency towards omnipotence. The patient's autistic part wants to transform reality to his own liking and avoid anguish by employing a narcissistic solution. Attempting to initiate an affective relationship will call for considerable strength and self-confidence on the part of the analyst. He has to fight against the imposition of a passive role that the patient wants to attribute to him. Moreover, the analyst must also recognize any possible collusion of his own with the patient's projections.

Faced with such situations, the problem is to maintain a balance between emotional closeness with the patient, a closeness which is good enough to allow the analyst to stay in touch with the suffering part, which will be full of damage and despair, and at the same time maintain a distance that allows us to consider how to deal with the difficulties of listening and finding meaning in the different neurotic and psychotic parts of the patient. The processing function operating between these parts can only be activated when the analytic relationship is strengthened.

The problem is how to help the patient begin thinking. The continuing effort will be to re-join two mental functions in the patient's mind, since primitive emotional experiences have been excluded from the Ego up to that point. It will be important to make such feelings recognizable, and to make connections between feelings and thoughts. This can be done by using the material produced by the patient and by providing for thinking about the manifold meanings contained in it, in such a way that the patient can discover the multiplicity of thoughts. The analyst should therefore become aware of her own feelings, keep them inside and think of possible interventions only according to the patient's current level of integration.

At this stage, the thought has to become thinkable in ourselves before giving it to the patient through interpretations. Bion (1979) suggests the necessity of taking all the time that may be required because the patient's current experience has to be carefully explored. This allows the analyst to give shape and meaning to his thoughts.

Regarding the development of thinking, Bion (1967) emphasizes the importance of paying attention and asking questions so that preconceptions are understood. He also suggests that the analyst give a name to things in order to tie them together so that they do not go astray, and that the meaning of a set of ideas be allowed to develop naturally and gradually. The development of meanings can unfold when preconceptions and their realization may proceed (at the same time) within the analytic relationship. Thoughts can then grow as previously 'unsaturated' elements and thus can be appropriately acknowledged. Through the process of interpersonal interacting and the developing bond between patient and analyst, the great number of meanings evident in the patient's material hopefully leads to the development of thinking.

During the phase when the therapist tries to take on and develop meaningful significances, there will be incidences when certain patients may present the analyst with a difficulty. While carrying out apparently intellectual activities in confronting examples and new associative hypotheses, such patients may ask the therapist to repeat what he has said and even ask for further explanations because 'they didn't understand'. What can be noted here is the partial chronic deficiency in the process of symbolization, as well as difficulty in accepting novelty or understanding metaphors.

A frequent problem is a great interest in repeating the same subject. (see 'chuntering', Joseph, 1982) In other cases, a 'wall of words' may be built as an intellectual autistic barrier rather than be used for real communication.

The lack of symbolization is also evident in dreams: when some patients begin to dream they don't associate anything to their dreams, and cannot find meaning in the story the dream tells. The dreams are considered only as a set of facts and are recounted as if they were descriptions of photographs, just as an action is perceived by bodily sensations, felt to be real, but unconnected to possible meanings, conscious or unconscious.

The patient's dreams allow the analyst to work at attributing and amplifying the meanings of the actions within them, and to explore the feelings of the dream characters. Sometimes, however, dreams are 'thrown' into the consulting room like closed packages with unknown contents, only produced in order to demonstrate obedience to formal analytic rules.

Faced with the void of the patient's thinking, I had to provide several associations of my own, according to my way of feeling and thinking at that time about the details or facts told to me. I did this in order to offer a range of thoughts and/or hypotheses, which were previously 'unknown' in the patient's mind. In this way, the patient can choose among many meanings to find the one he finds most relevant and assign a personal meaning to the dream, thus widening his own particular way of thinking.

Klein (1957) points out that, if feelings and meanings are not present in the communication, 'we cannot translate unconscious elements into conscious ones without lending our own conscious realm to the project'.

Another consequence of the absence of symbolization will surround the apparent lack of understanding and acceptance of the rules of the setting. Some patients would arrive with varying delays of up to half an hour, thus reducing the work time and controlling the waiting analyst. This same behaviour would occur regarding payment for the sessions. As I have emphasized previously, with neurotic patients we might interpret these delays, but in these cases, this kind of interpretation would be premature and inappropriate. My attempts to offer meaning when faced by these repetitive behaviours were useless. The problem was that the concept of time was absent as an internal coordinate of the Self.

In these cases, containment can be difficult because this strange behaviour interferes with the continuation of the analytical work, as well as its essential rules. As the analysis progressed, when the affective relationship was established, these same patients would finally be punctual and recognize the thoughtlessness embedded in their previous delays.

The continuous variation in the level of the patient's communication and of the resulting countertransference can be disturbing and confusing for the analyst. A safe compass for the analyst in such cases will be that of his own emotional reaction, felt immediately, even before he begins to think about the meaning of these messages. This reaction will be analysed and used to further process the material provided by the patient.

In the case of patients with addiction to drugs, alcohol, sex and gambling, an easy escape route from the analytic field will emerge through acting-out. It is difficult to eliminate this kind of resistance because in the past such behaviour represented a safe haven, an escape from the thinking Self, as in the case of those possessing internal autistic objects.

Making progress in the analysis is difficult because it represents the beginning of a separation, and separation is frightening. The realization that one has built a false identity over the years and the vision of a new picture of oneself as a person with his or her own humanity and mistakes will arouse feelings of depression in the patient. The difficulty will be in becoming aware that one's past self-confidence was based on arrogance and omnipotence.

At this point, the deflation of the personality, from an idealized omnipotent position to the perception of one's own real weakness, must be accompanied by tact and closeness on the part of the analyst, taking into account the patient's previous experience of existential emptiness.

During this process, the idealization of the analyst might also be an important temporary step towards the identification of their own capacity to think and to take into consideration hostility towards internal objects (Alvarez, 1992).

During this phase of the analysis, taking her cue from a film about how different scientific stimuli can lead to different results in scientific experiments, Sara is thrilled to discover that she herself can choose from a range of meanings and thoughts, and that these can be used to formulate a hypothesis in terms of future personal projects. What becomes manifest is a new idea of identity and responsibility.

At the descriptive level, the work helps these patients really experience and understand their feelings, and explore the various meanings of their relationships, before they can become engaged in the processes of introjection, internalization and identification.

Third: explanatory level

The explanatory level can be adopted when the interpersonal relationship is consolidated and we can begin to interpret the content and transference. This will allow the patient's personality to develop.

According to Alvarez, the explanatory level is the one where the analyst provides different meanings alongside interpretations, emphasizing the bond between the different parts of the personality, recognizing the projected parts seen in others, and transforming unconscious elements into conscious ones. This work makes it possible to allow the overall development of the patient's personality by using the analytical tool of interpretation.

The patient will accept interpretations of the transference when his or her identity is more solid and the process of separation is acknowledged.

At this point, the deflation of the personality from an idealized, omnipotent image to one where there is a perception of weakness must be accompanied by the analyst's attentive listening and empathic awareness, bearing in mind how easy one can resort to former states of emptiness.

When the analytic relationship is kept alive for a long period of time, despite misunderstandings, moments of stalemate and development, gradually a new way of thinking emerges, which is fertile and open to future developments. At that point, it is possible to imagine coming closer to an end.

As Ogden (2003) points out, psychological development can occur if one is able to accept the fact that primitive experiences can neither be modified nor transformed into those we would desire. Reaching this development through analysis is impossible since it is impossible to break the unconscious bond of contempt, anger and disappointment experienced at a very early stage.

12.2 Discussing the ending

Talking about the end after these long therapeutic journeys together is difficult for both patient and analyst because of the complexity of communication which comes back into mind. The darkness of unexplored internal spaces re-emerges, along with the fluctuations of emotional experiences and the difficulties faced in the encounter.

At the end of the phase of interpretation, it is important to plan for a period in which the final separation can be processed, as this is an emotionally significant moment. Separation brings up fantasies and dreams that can enrich the new experience by acknowledging that an affective bond between two people has developed over time and persists in the minds of each individual.

As with any affective relationship, separating is painful for both. In some patients, proposing a period to process the end is met with rejection, perhaps because of an unconscious fear that separating will be as painful as it was in the their past. However, that means that it is still difficult to share a thought, a project with someone else, without losing our individuality.

Analysis is thus interrupted with an arbitrary motivation, which varies from person to person, because they cannot face the meaning of the word 'conclusion'.

In the fortunate case where both patient and analyst recognize that there has been an evolution in the Self of the patient towards a new and creative way of life, and that the initial symptoms have been overcome, the imminent separation will represent another experience of the loss of the original absent object. At the same time, new feelings of love and the inevitable ambivalence towards the original objects will also be experienced.

In hindsight, when the end comes, one can consider that the emergence of a disintegrative crisis, which in these cases may have started off an analysis in a dramatic way, can be reassuring in that the subject now acknowledges a need for an authentic Self. When the mask is broken, the feelings that had previously been excluded can be retrieved. The states of disintegration can constitute a starting point in the search for a more integrated sense of Self. This new Self will allow greater security in that the subject can acknowledge within himself the various parts that had been expelled and projected onto the other, as well as accepting and integrating the various transition phases of mental development, paranoid-schizoid and depressive.

Thus, the polarization towards the negative characteristics of primitive objects, and the need to make claims and accusations for what occurred during childhood, fade as the person attempts to become an individual with personal characteristics, replacing false defences with their own truth.

12.3 Technique or analytic style?

The word 'technique' derives from the Greek (tèchne). It signifies art in the sense of skill, knowing one's job and knowing how to act and represent a set of norms, applied as both a manual and an intellectual activity.

In psychoanalysis, this set of norms is represented by psychoanalytic theories, by the experiences handed down by those who have preceded us, by recent studies, and last but not least, by our own feelings in encounters with a specific patient.

In training groups held by Resnik in Venice starting in the 1970s, he compared the process of the analyst's learning to that which took place in the ateliers of artists during the Italian Renaissance. Through the continuity of interactions, pupils and masters got to know each other, and communication could take place in a common area that allowed for exchange, differentiation and the exercise of new intuitions, until the individual artist could differentiate himself from a background of technical knowledge learned from others and develop his own particular style.

I think that the style of the analyst will change over the course of time, in every single case and in every single phase. It is revealed at the exact moment when the stimuli dictated by an encounter with the individual patient intertwine with the peculiar elements of the analyst's own experience and personality. Style cannot therefore be codified in norms, or reproduced. Encounters with those who are acknowledged as 'masters' in the art and science of psychoanalysis is formative because of the direct experience with the person-analyst and his specific way of working, which cannot be imitated. This can help our own preconceptions in the formation of new thoughts.

Introducing a study regarding the main features of Bion's work, Ogden (2003, 2007) specifies that one speaks of analytic technique when referring to a set of norms shared by analysts, both those working in the past and those working now. In contrast, if one speaks of 'analytic style', they refer to the work of a single analyst who will possess his or her own personality and experience, which cannot be reduced to a set of precisely followed norms, valid for everyone. In 'analytic style', not everything an analyst does will be 'analytic'; and the ways he behaves in sessions will also not only be personal. The analytic style is based on the analyst's particular personality: the particular way he uses his personal experience, as analyst and as analysand, as a child, son, parent, husband, wife, friend, teacher, student, etc. It is also based on his ability to remember the classic theories or those of his own analytic school, and be able to put them to one side, ultimately taking on personal responsibility for creating new ways of intervening.

12.4 Countertransference as a tool for therapeutic work

> What is the role of the mirror? To reflect what is before it. If no one is observing the mirror, does the mirror exist? The answer is no, because the

mirror exists only in the gaze and in the thought of the person who observes it. The function of the mirror cannot be separated from reflexive reasoning. The mirror reflects you and exists because you reflect yourself in it. Only an exercise in thought can make the mirror work. The mirror exists only if you recognise yourself in it. The mirror is an optical prosthesis used by the brain to understand and wonder about itself.

(Pistoletto, 2017)

There have been many studies regarding the countertransference as a crucial tool in analytic work. Since therapeutic work has been extended to include infantile autism and psychoses, countertransference has come back to the very centre of analytic work. It has also posed many questions regarding its practical uses and implementation.

By the term countertransference we usually mean the variety of feelings the analyst experiences in response to the transference, and which he needs to process and then feed back in a form that is acceptable to the patient. In the case of patients who are experiencing a crisis of dissolution of the Self, one may wonder what kind of communication can take place in the transference, considering that the patient is communicating fears or existential terrors but cannot express them symbolically. So the analyst feels that his method of working is threatened by the impossibility of communicating, and he feels powerless and alone.

This leads to a search for similar states in the labyrinth of one's subconscious, or for a ray of intuition that can grant greater serenity, as far as one is able to, within the analytical space. To move forward with the work, the analyst must search within himself to connect his emotions to comprehensible words and look for associations within himself, standing in for the patient.

Failure in this task, or the weakness of the patient's representations of the primary object, along with a lack of instinctual satisfaction due to the dearth of affective exchanges, will result in emotional withdrawal and cannot be expressed through language.

We must therefore resign ourselves to this persistent wish to search for personal meanings, but give up the usual methods of therapeutic intervention. We must accept that we do not know how to proceed in a way that is useful to the patient. The attempts to make this encounter effective thus become both personal and arbitrary, raising theoretical questions.

Hence, analytic work specifically with patients with autism, whether children or adults, will draw on connections with different degrees of personal sensitivity, our personal histories of emotional development and our identifications. The recognition of this personal analytic journey allows more freedom of expression with the patient, giving authenticity to the work, and establishing a strong continuity in the relationship, which goes beyond specific theories.

Maybe our tolerance and patience when faced with the attacks of the patient against his therapy and our difficulty in understanding this will depend on the tolerance and patience that our parents and grandparents had towards our own immature and youthful behaviour.

David Rosenfeld (2006) pointed out that therapeutic feelings that emerge in these cases are influenced more by our own affective and emotional background than by classical theories and analytical training. He admits having learned more from his relationship with his grandmother than from psychoanalytic theories. This led him to build a model where the analyst is capable of listening, understanding and thinking, giving respect to a fellow human being who talks about his own life and his feelings.

I would like to conclude by recalling the concept of double transference (as opposed to that of countertransference) introduced by Resnik (1972) to signify a double transmission of messages. If the analyst simultaneously takes on the position of analyst as well as that of patient, he or she can relate to what the patient transmits as well as to his or her own regressive nuclei and identificatory processes.

Thus, Resnik talks about the exchange in this 'double transference' referring to the 'theory of the gift'. According to anthropologists (Mauss, 1923; Malinowski, 1979), the archaic gift demonstrates a relational totality in a community built around the circulation of gifts and counter-gifts.

Berthoud (1991) thinks that a gift is a complex phenomenon, especially in its most ancient form, that of a total service.

> Souls get mixed up with things; things get mixed up with souls. Lives intermix and this is how people and things, mixed together, each come out of their own sphere and are mixed up: this is nothing more than a contract and an exchange. Exchanges don't involve single individuals, but an entire collectivity.
>
> Things that are exchanged are never completely detached from their exchanger ... the thing itself is not inert. Although it may be abandoned by the giver, it still retains something of his own spirit. In Maori law, the legal constraint, the constraint through things, is a bond between souls, because the thing in itself has a soul, it belongs to the soul. And this is how giving something to someone is equivalent to giving something of oneself...; accepting something from someone is equivalent to accepting something of their spiritual essence, of their soul..., there is, first of all, a mixing of spiritual bonds between things, individuals and groups.
>
> (Mauss, 1923)

12.5 Final reflections: why do some patients remain longer in our minds than others?

The analyst welcomes, with the same careful listening, emotional requests made by patients through projective identification, but in clinical practice our experience is that some patients occupy our mind more intensely than others between sessions. Why is this?

This may be owing to several factors. The most obvious of these is the knowledge that the person's physical and mental life is in serious danger.

In the event that a patient manifests suicidal thoughts, or a high degree of regression with experiences of abandonment, our attention and concern are present beyond the sessions and may also require our action: we must intervene and provide concrete urgent help when we feel there is a need. I believe that in these cases one must pull away from the neutrality prescribed by classical psychoanalysis, to be more responsive to the needs and the fragility of the patient.

In the case of a depressed patient or one who is recovering from a crisis of depersonalization, the analyst who must take a leave of absence for personal or business reasons may feel the need to make a phone call to transmit by voice the continuity of the relationship, especially if the concept of absence has not yet been processed. Nevertheless, being close in thought, even between sessions, already constitutes a therapeutic factor.

If a patient brings a recent experience of severe psychic or physical trauma to the session, the analyst has to deal with her/his own ability/inability to internally process such a tragic occurrence.

In my experience with patients who have suffered early trauma, the transference/countertransference relationship has required a lot of effort to get out of the prevailing world of psychic death. The early onset and the violence of the initial trauma, indicated by the patient's history and perceived through our countertransference, contribute to our mentally taking care of that patient in a more continuous way than we would with others. Excessive identification with one's own experiences can also foster permanence in one's mind.

Conversely, the analyst often has a particular patient in mind when that particular subject has psychopathic traits, is very irritating or places many obstacles in the way of establishing a collaborative relationship; or when the patient poses a physical threat and therefore evokes feelings of fear. In this case, the analyst's mind is filled with pressing issues: the presence of sadistic personal feelings evoked by the other; how to tolerate a disturbing atmosphere; how to proceed and eliminate destructive feelings; how to escape constant manipulation and how to transform the wishes of discharge into productive interventions.

Patients who are more present in our memories for long periods of time, even after the end of analysis, can remain so because they had such a profound change in their internal states and were the witnesses of a fertile and intense human relationship.

Though it may be unexpressed or unknown, the help that the patient needs in analysis is that of being present in the mind of the other as a representative of valid support. The patient wishes to have someone who thinks about her/him, who understands those moments that are unbearable for her/him, so that she/he may internalize an understanding and supportive object that can allow him to exist as an individual.

In terms of borderline psychopathology, Gerald Adler (1977, 1988; Adler and Buie, 1979), stated that some patients have a fear of feeling alone without an internal support.

Goldberg (2015) emphasizes that the analyst, too, needs the presence of patients in his mind, in that they represent the world in which he has chosen to live and work. In fact, we must not forget that in offering ourselves as therapists we try in turn to be present in the minds of others and to cultivate human relations. If the relationship with a patient is characterized by harmony and creative intensity, the analyst feels a general sense of well-being. On the other hand, if excessive self-assurances, on both sides, clash and attempt to prevail, the sense of unease carries on even beyond the sessions and the failure of the encounter.

References

Adler, G. (1977) *Borderline psychopathology and its treatment*, New York: Jason Aronson.
Adler, G. (1988) 'How useful is the borderline concept?', *Psychoanalytic Inquiry*, 8, 353–372.
Adler, G. and Buie, D. (1979) 'Aloneness and borderline psychopathology', *International Journal of Psychoanalysis*, 60, 83–96.
Alvarez, A. (1980) 'Two regenerative situations in autism: reclamation and becoming vertebrate', *Journal of Child Psychotherapy*, 6(1), 69–80.
Alvarez, A. (1992) *Live company*, London and New York: Tavistock and Routledge.
Alvarez, A. (2012) *The thinking heart*, London and New York: Routledge.
Berthoud, G. (1991) 'Somlo et l'ordre généralisée du don' ('Somlo and the generalized regime of gift'), *La revue du Mauss* (nouv. ser. 14), 83–92.
Bick, E. (1968) 'The experience of the skin in early object-relations'. In A. Briggs (ed.) *Surviving space: papers on infant observation* (pp. 55–59), London: Karnac, Tavistock Clinic Series, 2002.
Bion, W. R. (1958) 'On arrogance', *International Journal of Psychoanalysis*, 39, 266.
Bion, W. R. (1967) *Second thoughts: selected papers on psychoanalysis*, London: Heinemann.
Bion, W. R. (1979) 'Making the best of a bad job'. In *Clinical seminars and other works* (pp. 321–323), London: Karnac.
Bowlby, J. (1979) *The making and breaking of affectional bonds*, London: Tavistock Publications.
Goldberg, A. (2015) *The brain, the mind and the self*, London: Routledge.
Houzel, D. (2001) 'Bisexual qualities of the psychic envelope'. In J. Edwards (ed.), *Being alive: building on the work of Anne Alvarez* (pp. 44–56), Hove: Brunner-Routledge.
Joseph, B. (1982) 'Addiction to near-death'. In E. B. Spillius and M. Feldman (eds), *Psychic equilibrium and psychic change: selected papers of Betty Josef* (pp. 127–138), London: Routledge, 1989.
Klein, M. (1957) 'Envy and gratitude'. In *The writings of Melanie Klein, volume III* (pp. 176–235), London: Hogarth, 1975.
Malinowski, B. (1979) *The ethnography of Malinowski: the Trobriand Islands 1915–18*, London: Routledge & Kegan Paul.

Mauss, M. (1923) 'Essai sur le don. Forme et raison de l'échange dans les sociétés archaiques'. In *Sociologie ET anthropologie* (pp. 145–279), Paris: PUF, nuoniva ed., 1985.

Ogden, T. H. (2003) 'On not being able to dream: essays', *International Journal of Psychoanalysis*, 84(1), 17–30.

Ogden, T. H. (2007) 'Elements of analytic style: Bion's clinical seminars', *International Journal of Psychoanalysis*, 88, 1185–1200.

Pistoletto M. (2017) *Omniteismo e demopraxia*, Milano: Chiarelettere Editore.

Resnik, S. (1972) *Personne e psychose*, Paris: Editions du Hublot.

Rosenfeld, D. (2006) *The soul, the mind and the psychoanalyst*, London: Karnac.

Conclusions

This book bears witness to the analytic journeys taken in search of autistic (pre-mental) states responsible for disorders in the psychic economy of adult patients. The experiences that have conditioned the development of the Self are often hidden behind neurotic, borderline or psychotic structures. The initial difficulty lies in recognizing the mask that the patient has constructed over the years to avoid and hide from primitive suffering.

The ability to identify these unrepresented states through analysis takes place mainly through the countertransference. In the initial contact, the analyst is aware of the lack of immediate feelings, which are normally indispensable to establish a therapeutic alliance. Thus the fundamental tool to approach these primitive painful areas rests precisely on the countertransference.

Following emotionally significant events, these hidden experiences may manifest through acute crises of disintegration of the Self. When faced with a patient's experience of existential terror, the analyst must first of all try to come into contact with the patient, as well as with his own primitive world in order to be able to translate emotions into words. He must also try to welcome the patient's fragments, acknowledge the unprocessed elements in search of meaning and decipher their physical signs in order to subsequently transform these symbolically.

This book also contains reflections on the interconnections between non-represented mental states and the functions of the skin as a container and primitive organ of communication with the outside world. By paying constant attention to the patient's body, one can obtain invaluable information about emotional history, because the body is the living memory of primitive experiences.

The process of the patient becoming aware of these experiences and understanding their influence on the development of his personality takes several years. Recognizing one's true Self forces visions and false certainties of the past to shift, and these shifts require some time to settle before life can be given to a new Self.

From a therapeutic standpoint, it is difficult to regulate the distance between patient and analyst: owing to primitive experiences of early shortcomings, the patient may tend towards fusion or con-fusion. At the same time, however, proximity may be seen as intrusion. Being two people *without* fusion means respecting the space between oneself and the other, accepting differences and maintaining contact through an affective bond. Thus, the shortcomings of the primitive bond re-emerge.

It is very important to pay attention to the fluctuations of one's own feelings and intuitions and to conduct continuous self-analysis. All this allows the patient's identity to develop and change, and leads to new therapeutic reflections on oneself.

The containing function of the analyst does not always find useful creative elements to offer the patient, and this failure can be a source of pain and anxiety for both. Only the therapist's plasticity will allow continuous adaptations to variations in the transference, modulating the type of intervention depending on the moment and the phases of the development of the relationship. In this way, the relationship will develop through continuous monitoring of the transference–countertransference exchange.

Index

abandonment fear of 12; experiences of 151; feelings of 28; physical distance as a form of 75; processing experience of 27; threat of 15

acting-out/actings-out 10, 60, 85, 122; conveys inability to express aggressive feelings 73; evasion through 127; interpreting 65; patients with addictions 135, 145; persistent 56; repeated 80; separation followed by 135

addiction(s) 12, 77, 85, 135, 145; accepted 104; to bad affective experiences 136; development of 127; drug 57, 62, 73; external turn to 134; to a past close to psychic death 110; to sensory experiences 55; sex 56, 62, 66, 90, 135–136; to violence 60

addictive: love 108; solution 90

adhesive: analytic relationship 59; attachments 75, 95; autistic children 125; bonds 15; mode of being 36; proximity 74; second skin 41

adhesive identification 35–36, 41, 124; excessive process of 44

adhesiveness 59, 77, 97

adhesive relationship 122; without space for communication 89

Adler, G. 152

adult patients 1; with autistic mental states 120; with autistic nuclei 138; with autistic residues 129; borderline psychological structure 8; classic analytical approach 142; difficulties in taking up classical analytical work 10; disorders in the psychic economy of 154; hiding a regressive part 84; non-represented states 11; with traces of autism 7

aesthetic impact of child on maternal reality 44; importance of 44; paralyzing 45; reciprocity of 43

affective relationship(s) 86, 145; adult, primitive relationships at the root of 108; allow preconceptions to turn into thoughts 100; attempting to initiate 143; autistic nuclei that lie far from 2; autistic structure that prevented 95; conclusion of analytic work around 106; defence in by various forms of addiction 127; difficulty in lack of continuity of feelings 104; personal dilemma regarding 102; primitive sensory experiences 84; profound 81; reduced 10; separating is painful for both 147; stability impossible 108; strengthened 135; success attributed to number of partners 136

aggression 142; acceptance of 99; affectionate feelings replaced by 92; awareness of own 70; in dreams 70, 75–76; feeling not recognized as something personal 119; in first contact 117; shown in repeated behaviours 64; towards others 61; towards the Self 28; in transference 77, 135; trying to contain patient's 96, 99

aggressive 59; behaviour 96; destructive return of projected material 28; forces 83; gestures, respond to 84; outbursts targeted at self 45; tool 72; verbally 86; way of communicating 60

aggressive attacks 56; on own body 61; targeted at self 45

aggressive feelings 45; denial of 10; inability to express 73

aggressiveness 79, 104; archaic 106;

Index   157

difficult to contain 57; patient's 83; perceived 128; volume 119
Aisenstein, M. 21n1
allergic: conjunctivitis 60; reactions 29–30, 87–88; *see also* eczema
allergies 30, 60
Alvarez, A. 10, 35, 64, 77, 80, 82, 85, 96, 124–126, 128, 138, 142, 146
amplification/amplifying 142, 145
analytical 129, 141; classic approach with adult patients 142; couple 133; disempowerment, attempt at 111; experiences of the present 136; listening 10; process 125; space 149; tool of interpretation 146; training 150
analytical relationship 142; communication in 7; effort to stay in 122; important to move forward with courage 128; lack of pudore in 126; must have a guide 127; turns into state of helplessness and suffering 123
analytical thinking 133; obstacle to development of 127
analytical work 7, 126; classical 10; with contiguous-autistic or paranoid-schizoid mental states 134; controlling behaviour of patient interferes with continuation 145; patient attempts to prove no benefit from 124; reaching deep levels of disintegration 133
annihilation 14; anxiety 13
anthropologist(s) 16, 150
Anzieu, D. 15, 21n2, 31–32
Anzieu-Premmereur, C. 21n2
armour 52–53, 87; anonymous 98; autistic 29, 32; cardboard 98; defensive, abandoned 29; entrenched/enclosed in 1–2, 9; maintaining 20; of others, attempt to penetrate 20; represented in various ways 134; wearing objects of great value as 27
Artaud, A. 52
at first sight: immediate sensory experiences 46; love 39; love or hate 39
autism 1–2, 36, 45, 94, 122, 138; in adults 126; analytic work in patients with 149; in children 7, 10, 29, 34, 40, 126, 134; defensive manoeuvres of patients 127; immobility in interpersonal relationships 143; infantile 149; obsessive defences 136; perverse mechanisms 135; skin and body image in 28–29, 34; two-dimensional mental functioning 35; underlying psychotic symptomatology 99
autistic 1, 7; activities (bodily sensations) 62, 73; armour 29, 32; barrier 144; manoeuvres, repetitive 134; mental states 41, 120; modalities 127; nucleus/nuclei 2, 7, 11, 18, 63, 86, 103, 134–136, 138; objects 9, 46, 60, 95, 104, 135, 145; part 143; parts hidden 126; patients 88, 124, 139; primitive reactions 8; refuge, loss of 87; residues 53, 109, 126, 129; shapes 62, 66; space 20; states 3, 54; structure 95; subjects 125; traces 38; type capsules 8; withdrawal 89, 101; world 40, 88
autistic children 13; armour, protective 29; avoidance of eye contact 119; bodily sensations 65, 92n1; experience moments of terror 29; loss of Ego 125; sensitive qualities of surfaces 40; *see also* children with autism
autistic-contiguous/contiguous-autistic 34; mental states 134; primitive experience 40
autistic experiences 9, 65, 97; of moments of crisis 123; sensory 18; prevails 87, 96; primitive 3, 136; transference in patients 121
autistic object(s) 95, 135; analyst as 125, 134; attempt to transform a person into 60, 123; internal 145; words as 9, 104
autistic states 154; emptiness of 123; experiences of 3, 7; narcissism of 142; reflect on 54; separation from 86

Barrows, K. 1, 7
beautiful 27, 38, 42, 71; connected to fetishism 70; judged to be 43; people and things 41; scissors 77; skin 68; women 43–44
beauty 41–44, 71; concept of 53; crucial experiences of 46; immediately perceived 38; lack of 45
Bergstein, A. 124
Berthoud, G. 150
Bick, E. 28–29, 32–33, 35–36, 41, 64, 139
Bion, B.W. 133
Bion, W. 3, 8, 10, 12–13, 46, 56, 80–81, 87, 100, 125, 143–144, 148
black hole(s) 8, 13–14, 21n3, 63, 66, 75, 79
bodily 140, 143; care of the child 34; dissolution, crisis of 87; excitement masking real feelings 140; fluids 29;

Index

bodily *continued*
  forms, lack of standard 45; functions, child's 33; message given by patient 125; movements 140; organ (skin) 55; products 27; sense of being 'one' 33; sensory perceptions 41; sign 61; signs of communication 82; surface of the child 41 tension 12
bodily behaviour 138, 140; of drug addicts 61
bodily contact, need for 62; contacts, close 74; disintegration, fear of 67; dissolution, crisis of 66; experiences, early 76; experiences as forms of contact 66; image 66; limits, absence of 82; organ 67; separation 66; states, description of 74; symptoms, new 63
bodily experiences 41; of emptiness 90; primitive 32; of suffering 87
bodily sensations 29; action is perceived by 145; of autistic child 92; employed to avoid a vacuum 135; experienced 61; fundamental in establishing identity 66; primitive states of 29; repetition of autistic activities 62
body/bodily image 3; in autism 28–29; autistic experiences in 65; compared to sheet of paper 88; development of 29; difficulties with 134; disorder of 67; one's own representation of 18; primitive 31; sensory couplings in 66
body language 60, 120
Botella, C. 13, 21n2
Bowlby, J. 15–16, 142
breakdown: mental, fear of 8; psychotic 1

Calvino, I. 52–53
Cassoria, R.M. 21n2
childhood 70, 103; defensive barriers 126; emotional states of suffering 12; family environment 105; feelings of rejection or degradation 110; omnipotence as defence in 76
childhood experiences 2, 105, 147; of being patient 132; of catastrophe in psychotics 13; of direct contact 17; having to acknowledge and process 29; lack of emotional security 16; physical and emotional 3; representation of 43; sensory, unprocessed 8; un-mentalized 55
children 103; anxiety experienced by 15; in dreams 67–68, 70; immediate reaction to new encounters 39; inability to raise her own 109; mother/children relationship 111; primitive bad experiences 125; with psychosis or drug addiction 57; psychotic traits 80; taking care of 98; unable to symbolize what has not been experienced 96
children with autism 134; adhere to sensitive qualities of surfaces 40; clinical work with 10; damaged Self and internal objects 138; feeling states frozen within 96; image of the body 29; lost parts of the Ego 125; moments of terror/nameless dread experienced 8, 29; psychoanalytic work with 2; second skin constructed 29; therapy with 126; treatment with 138; unable to establish an object relationship 96
chuntering *see* repeat/repeated/repeating same subject
Civitarese, G. 7, 21n2
countertransference 1–2, 7, 9, 74, 96, 110, 150–151; analysing 55; analysis of progression 129; analyst experiences 129–130; analyst's discomfort in 142; continuous monitoring of 155; dangers in feelings of 128; difficult to deal with 109; experience 53, 120, 126; fluctuations in 60, 80, 104, 122; narcissistic 80; negative 57; process 54, 112, 120, 127; thoughts and feelings shared 121; tool for therapeutic work 10, 148–149, 154; ups and downs of 126; variability of 126; variations confusing for analyst 145
Cremerius, J. 65

death 66, 76; absence of intercourse led to 62; anxiety about 138; brought on depression 103; in dreams 69, 71, 75; drive 11; emotional 130; in family 103, 105; instinct 13; internal 125, 129; life confused with 40, 96; mental 124; mother's love can lead to feelings of death 107; phantasies about 95; psychic 110, 151; separation experienced as patient's own 135, 143; of stars 21n3; thinking about 63; world of 75
death, fear of 13; of loss linked to 122
death, imminent 68; psychic 107
deathly: atmosphere 75; feelings 73
death of Self 90; of meanings of Self 13
depersonalization, crisis of 67, 94, 151

depressed: analyst 122; children 77; mother 130; patient 123, 151
depression 13, 114; analyst attempts to escape 112; autistic manoeuvres used to avoid 134; development of latent 130; feelings of 141, 146; of mother 103; narcissistic 84; no moment of 59; projected onto analyst 128; retreat into 12; unable to acknowledge 103
depressive: anxieties 114; experience, first 66; functioning 18; position, development towards 91; state caused by analytic work 74; states 114
depressive feelings 90; analyst overcome by 58; devaluating other person to avoid falling into 71; experience of vacuum does not contain 136; triggered the onset of 84
depressive phase 147; assessment of past led to 79; autistic manoeuvres to avoid the shame of 134; emergence of 127; prevented by narcissism 84, 103; process of separation from autistic state to 86
désaffectés 3, 129
desperate 78; children 77; need of the exciting object (addictive love) 108
desperation 124–125
development 2–3, 15, 28, 45, 84, 106, 120; of ability to create differentiated symbols 20; in acknowledgement of behaviour 77; of addictions 127; of allergic disorders 30; of approach 142; of areas privileged for sexual functions 33; of body image 29; cultural 42; devoid of possible 122; differentiation and union 31; Ego 8, 110; emotional 18, 20, 141, 149; of events 132; of foetus, defects in 71; future 113, 146; hinder 52; no possibility of 123; over time 100–101; partial deficit in cognitive 57; personality 44, 126, 154; of primitive skin function, failure of 32; reached through analysis 147; stages of 21n3, 40; therapeutic 80, 99
development, affective 3; distance 17; primitive phases 96, 99
development of analytic work 35, 113; confidence in process 141; first period 64; previous session 71; thinking, obstacle to 127; of traditional analytic discourse 10

development, child's 18, 21; early 7, 13, 19, 21n1; lack of early support 36; normal 32; of process of symbolization 18
development of depressive position 91; of latent 130
development of meanings 144; mediated by the object 12
development, mental 3, 88; process 134; transition phases of 147
development, patient's 77; obstacle to 114; personality 146; psychic 101; psychological 147
development of process of symbolization: child's 18; defective 7, 18
development, psychic 26; apparatus 31; interior space 20; patient's 101
development of relationships 112; between skin and Self 26; parasite-host or *folie-à-deux* 28; phases of 155; prevented 120; therapeutic 99; transformed 46
development of the Self 88; hidden experiences conditioned 154; intervention appropriate for individual degree of 8; of one's own sense of 17; part strives for new 14; process of 9; relationship between the skin and 26; therapeutic relationship allows changes to arise that determine 99; time enriches 41; of undeveloped part of personality 84
development of space: concept of 15; defect in sense of internal space 36; interior psychic 20
development of thinking 11, 113, 144; in analysis 10; obstacles to analytical 127
disintegration 141; acute situations of 121; cases of 82; crisis of 28, 138; deep levels of 133; emergence from phase of 142; fear of 63; fear of bodily 67; of the individual 52; patient experiences state of 124; primitive experiences of 55; of Self, acute crises of 154; sense of 107; separation becomes equivalent to 17; signs of personality 8; states of 147; varying degrees of 124
dissolution 82; bodily 66, 87; crisis of 149; danger of 64; internal danger of 74; symptoms of 74
Docker-Drysdale, B. 96, 128
dream(s) 79, 103; abundance of 83; acknowledgement of behaviour 77; activities 106; after crisis 64; awareness of inner world 76; based on crime 106;

dream(s) *continued*
bloodthirsty and apocalyptic 68; body abnormality 67; body and skin 87; brought up by separation 147; of death and mummification 75; dehumanized aspects of 69; describe in detail 104; desire to kill 65; experience of non-being 75; first 90; full of terror 68; of going away from family 102; gradual changes in relationship 75; interpreting 91–92; issues highlighted in 122; lack of symbolization evident 144; of living in a world devoid of imperfections 41; material 70, 84; of my fantasies 46; objects seen in 140; patient/mother 67; patient's 7, 66, 106, 145; personal meaning assigned 145; production of 59, 64, 73; recurring themes 68; of rediscovering love 39; regarding desolation 64; relating to parasites 89; showing modifications in transference 78; about skin 71–72; unable to find foothold 82; unconscious constructs 120; violent content 69

eczema 29–30, 60–61, 123
Ego 33, 51, 107; auxiliary 99; committed to hiding profound internal truth 85–86; difficulty to construct space and maintain distance 15; language directed by 86; libidinal 108; mask of 70; parts need to be reclaimed 125; primitive emotional experiences excluded from 144; sieve or shell (skin) 18; strength of 47
Ego development 8, 110; damaged 110
Ego functions 32; functional deficits 20; loss of important 32
Ego-skin 32
empathic: ability of analyst 133; awareness of analyst 146; with hidden suffering parts 127; identification with the infant 56; patient becoming 112; sharing 142
empathy 19; analyst's 81, 112; develop feelings of 83; maintaining 114; natural 118; no natural 109; ordinary or enduring 112
emptiness 8, 11, 13, 33, 91, 130; of autistic states 123; bodily experiences of 90; centripetal pull into the void 66; desolate 54; existential 146; feelings of 53, 124; internal 73; of mind 138; of non-being Self 62; primitive experience of 124; psychic 124; recurring themes of 125; of thought 111; terror of 90; transition from a state of 142
erotic: contact point 31; eroticized orifices 62, 73
erotogenic experience 33; zone 61
Eshel, O. 14, 21n2
exhibition 9; of the body 126
exhibitionism 61

façade image 36
Fairbairn, W.R.D. 96, 106–108, 136
false Self 8, 52, 120
fantasy/fantasies 73; acknowledging masochistic tendency 111; about bodily products 27; of death and mummification 75; dream of 46; about expelling the patient 122; expressed through words 104; of fusion 74; maternal, internalization of 101; mind not capable of 35, 40; of non-mentalized world 66; offering 125; patient does not transmit 124; primitive 65, 74; repeating the same 91; separation brings up 147; sight leads to 119; of sharing skin with the mother 32; symbiotic 141; of termination 133
feelings 1–3, 9, 15, 17–18, 21, 28, 42–44, 46, 56, 75, 81, 86, 88, 114, 118, 121–122, 128–129, 133, 136, 140–141, 143; affection 62, 89, 92; of anxiety 63–64; blurred boundaries 67; conflicting 121, 126; contact 62, 80, 113; of dreams unaccompanied by 69; of loss of contact with reality 66; masked 140, 147; primitive 58, 110; processing 128; projection of 28; pudore 126; security 15, 62
feelings, absence/lack of 81, 100, 103, 110; affectionate 92; attachment 124; communication relating to 26; connection to 53; continuity 104; immediate 154; libido 107; profound 90
feelings of analyst 10, 128, 149; confronts deepest 124; in encounters with patients 148; evoked by the patient 128; inside 81; own 82, 144; relationship filled with 80; restores vitality with own 125; unconscious 80
feelings, bad 72; of abandonment 28, 68; of being excluded by mother 103; of being lost 133; of being made of air 123; of the body breaking into pieces 66; deathly 73; destructive 9, 91, 151; disappearing 35; of

disconnectedness and death 107; of disorientation 53, 59; of emptiness 53, 124; of falling into a black hole 13; fear of feeling alone 152; of guilt 58, 75; of impotence 80; of loneliness 63; out of place 38; pain/painful 41, 91, 113; paralyzed/frozen 12, 96, 104, 122; of persecution 96; of rejection or degradation 110; of strangeness 34; of suffering 28; of suspicion 39; of terror 29
feelings, communication 9, 112; absence of 26; blurred by language 60; centre of conversations 113; difficulty in expressing 66, 82; presence in 145; no space to debate 20; by sharing the same kind of 74
feelings, denying 113; of dependence 141
feelings of depression 58, 71, 84, 90, 136, 140–141; in patient 146; depressive feelings develop 34, 83; of empathy 83
feelings evoked 92n1, 127, 151; in analyst, by the patient 128; of disgust and death evoked 71; of fear 151
feelings, good 128; of being loved 130; of being in the presence 95; of being united with mother 36; of being welcomed 59; of gratitude 97; of pleasure 30; of satisfaction 12; of social inclusion 44
feelings of love 147; of being loved 130; continuity of 128; (and hate) towards therapist 121
feelings, negative: aggression/aggressive 10, 73, 119; anger 10, 100; contempt and rejection 104; of envy, greed and jealousy 42; hatred of psychotic part for feelings 128; hostility 61; violent, against self and against words 140
feelings of others 104; control of 123; deaf-mute 98; no mention of 26; patient did not care about 59, 89; understanding necessary in adult relationships 75; understood by pathological projective identification 16
feelings, own 77, 138; analyst's 82, 125, 144; fluctuations of 155
feelings of patient 33; depression 146; focus on being together 139; giving name to 84; help to understand 146; instability of 106; of more structured part of personality 142; no fluctuations of 71; of non-being/non-existence 73, 64; part far away from 83; personal 19; sadistic 151; of scarcity, persistent 136

feelings of power 136; sadistic 127, 151
feelings, protection from 64; armour for 9; defences against 129; fragmentation of 53
feelings, sharing 82, 112–113, 121; convergence of 140; passing from one to the other 41; same kind of 74
feelings and thoughts: connections with 144; linked 11; no connection 76
Ferenczi, S. 133
Fernandez, R. 26, 31
first encounters 9, 117
folie-à-deux relationships 28
Fonagy, P. 16, 83
fragmentation: anxiety about 138; attempt to overcome fear of 127; of the Ego 33; of relational experiences 136
Freud, S. 11, 18, 31, 33, 45, 51, 61
Freudian notion of bonding 16

gifts 117, 127; conciliatory 104; and counter-gifts 150
Goldberg, A. 112, 152
Green, A. 10–11, 20, 129–130
Groddeck, G. 51, 86
Grotstein, J.S. 8, 13–14, 20, 21n2, 66

Hall, E.T. 15–17
Hawking, S. 21n3
hole(s) 13; inside the body 29; in internal organs 33; in the stomach 63, 67; *see also* black hole(s)
hostility 3, 60; after bad affective experiences 136; feelings of 61; towards analyst 143; towards internal objects 146

idealization of analyst 146; of clothes or skin 27; necessary phase in patient's development 77; primitive 39
identification 119, 149; with different parts of internal objects 107; excessive 151; of own capacity to think 146; permanent, with rejecting parents 111; with sensations of familiar environment 139
identification adhesive 35–36, 41, 44, 124; as form of contact 31; with image given by other 34; initial forms of child's 31; intrusive 20; mimetic 18; with the mother 11; with object 31, 34; primitive processes of 35; unconscious 11; *see also* adhesive identification, projective identification(s)

identification with analyst 98; with a character made of wood 46; empathic, with infant 56; gender 79, 89; instinctive 39; male 67, 90; mimetic introjective 36; with patient 83; primitive, with 'It' 51; process impeded 94; sexual, problems with 74
identified: autistic-type capsules 8; with her child 83; with dead object 95, 138; as source of patient's relationship problems 109; unidentified corpses 69
identify/identifying 79; with abandoning object 28; with child-like aspects of patient's Self 81; connection with emotions experienced by patient 124; defences 141; failure 12; with need for help 142; with parts that need most attention 98; with patient's internal objects 122; parts of Self 1, 3; pathology 8; skin wounds, difficult 72; with rejecting object 108; unrepresented states 154
identity: confused 34; loss of 142
image(s) 67; abnormal 71; attempt to reproduce 67; of black hole 79; constructed 52; corresponds to visual representation 43; dreams made up of 70; existing beyond mental images 62; façade 36; failure to see connection to analysis 60; grandiose 59; idealized 146; identification with 34; internal 64; mental 32; mirror 39, 141; part of a chain of associations 81; of patient's life 38; patient's own 122; spatial 17; think through 81; of weakness and inability to think 123; of well-being and happiness 70
inertia 66, 90
introjection amplification will help 142; of containment object 31, 34; engage in processes of 146; impossible 83; made difficult 32; projective 28; regressive part has not reached the capacity of 84
Isaacs, S. 121
itching 30, 61; eyes 30, 60; represented bodily excitement 140

Keats, J. 47, 133
Khan, M. 21n2, 124
Klein, M. 145
Klein, S. 1, 7, 10, 18, 86, 134

language 11, 65, 118, 149; acquisition of 18; of affection, missing 110; aggressive 73; aimed at controlling analyst 104; analyst's 127, 140; body 60, 120; connected with identity and thinking 51; conveys messages 119; deaf-mute sign 98; disconnected from feelings 66; emotions too disturbing to translate into 121; expressed strange bodily sensations 29; foreign 97, 102, 117; Greek 52; inappropriate 56; lacking emotional depth 71; led to distortion of reality 80; more developed in adults 123; nuances of 127; precise 109; pudore 126; replaced with numbers 98; representation of objects through 133; of the skin 31; symbolic representation in 46; used by Ego to hide truth 85–86
Liberman, D. 15, 17–18, 35–36, 71
libidinal: Ego 108; level 33
libido, devoid of 107
love: backwards love 106; love at first sight 39, 46

Marty, P. 30
masked/masks: absence of self-worth 136; anxiety, by self-confidence 9; attack on the analyst 128; hidden autistic parts 126; inner truth 86; need for attachment 53; by projections 59; real feelings 140; by rejection of close relationships 15; rejection of real emotional contact 10; sadistic attacks 80; true Self 120
mask 27, 52; affective life separated from 85; of altruism 10; analyst 3; broken 147; clothes or make-up or hairstyle 119; collapsed 103, 105; communicate without 58; concealed confused identity 85; constructed over years 154; Ego 51, 70; hides the real face 52; importance of 70; misleading 89; needs coming from behind 82; of normality 1; outer 110; painful part hidden behind 55, 59; patient's, find truth beyond 53; protective defence 79; representing membership to social groups 27; social, removed 39; warrior 64; worn to adapt to normal life 102
masochistic: features 32; tendency 111
maternal 36, 102; adaptability in empathic identification 56; bond, primitive 74; closeness, absence of 89; environment 32; fantasies 101; functions 34; handling 33; internal world 43; protection 61; reality, aesthetic impact of child 44; reverie 56–57; situation 124; support 64, 142

Mauss, M. 150
McDougall, J. 3, 20, 30, 58, 86–87, 90, 129–130, 134
Meltzer, D. 20, 35–36, 39–41, 43–44, 88, 120
mentalization 16, 31, 73, 87
mentalized 66; experiences 14
Merleau-Ponty, M. 39
Mitrani, J. 7–8, 134
mother 63, 78, 97; absent 12, 90; alpha function 125; anxious 96; change in 99; clothes as substitute for body 27; dead 11, 27, 130; depressed 103, 130; discomfort reflected in 16; of the dream 67–68, 87–88; experience of motherhood 74; external 107; frustrations 106; gives affective meanings 62; grandmother 91, 150; inability to feel like 109; inaccessible 108; messages coming from 32; neglect on behalf of 14; personality disorder 19; phantasies about death of the foetus 95; psychotic 99, 104; reproducing conversation with 119; Self 43–44; verbal responses not asked for 124; *see also* maternal
mother and child: aesthetic impact on 44; attention and contact 35; breast 43–44; child's projections 13, 64; deficit of love for 106; limitations detected 106–107; perceived as object 19; physical discomfort felt/dealt with by 16; receptive to needs 36; space between 19; supporting 33; world introduced by 34
mother and child bond: difficulty in abandoning state of fusion with 30; ; early disconnection with 13; feeling of being united with 36; separation 15, 19; sharing skin with 32; terror of disconnection with 66
mother, child's relationship with 16–17, 43, 111; close, with sibling 89; difficult 103 identification, merging with 11, 66; primitive early experiences 125; unloving or unaccepting 107–108
mother, containing function 41; mental 41; child's projections 64

nameless dread 8, 13
narcissism 4, 90; analysis of 134, 141; of autistic states 142; aware of 79; destructive 122; feared the deflation of 75; obstacle to development of thought in analysis 10; prevented from reaching depressive phase 84; relinquishing 89; unfounded 134
narcissistic 27, 84; barrier 111; construction of personality 79; countertransference, defensive 80; defences 89; denial of presence 135; element 127; experience 39; homeostasis 45; injury 57; level 33; mirroring 43; need to win 128; organization 74; protective function 34; reinforcement 32; solution to avoid anguish 143; structure 65; wound 91, 103
negative capability 47, 133
new Self 147, 154
non-existence 8, 13; feeling came back 64; sense of 67; *The non-existent knight* 52
non-existent other: by avoiding eye contact 119; sessions 97
non-existent Self 64; partial 60
non-mentalized/unmentalized childhood experiences 55; experiences 8; nuclei 1; parts, difficulty of recognizing 86; primitive states 10; world filled with primitive sensations 66
non-represented material 7; mental states 10–11, 154; states 11, 13, 21n1

object relationship 40, 62; with allergic objects 30; characterized by lack of interest and attention 44; children unable to establish 96; emerging from symbiotic fusion 62; establishment of 11; existed only in the presence of the other 74; implied by apparent normality 84; internal 107; lack of 124; patient's primitive experience of 122; pudore is connected to 127; two-dimensional 41
Ogden, T.H. 7, 10, 19, 34–35, 40, 57–58, 106, 147–148
orifices 31, 40, 62, 73
own Self: birth of 44; communicative signs resonate in patient's 140; knowledge of, becomes more complete 52; task of 'I' to hide the truth from 51

parasite(s) 89; parasite-host relationship 28
Perrault, C. 27
phantasy/phantasies 32, 105; of baby to fill emptiness 91; of being excluded 95; of common skin with mother 32; about corpses 103; create 100; about dead parts of self 105; of death and crime 105; about the death of the foetus 95;

phantasy/phantasies *continued*
of envelope-container of internal organs 33; of external and internal space 31, 34; hypochondriac 91, 102; of merging with another 62; persecutory 97; rupture of abdominal skin 28; of skin with secondary containing function 41; unconscious 121; *see also* fantasy/fantasies
Pichon-Rivière, E. 30, 61
Pistoletto, M. 148–149
primitive experience(s) 1, 9, 13–14; absence of maternal closeness 89; adult patient relives 139; autistic 3; of being unable to keep any external element 'outside' 67; body is living memory of 154; children who have had 125; of disintegration 55; of early shortcomings 154; of emotional solitude 79; of emptiness 124; fought with reactions of mania and omnipotence 128; of the 'It' beyond the Self 51; mental construction based on 121; of object relationship 122; personal areas of 81; two-dimensional 124; unable to move away from 76
primitive experience(s) of the skin 18, 72; autistic-contiguous, originating from 40
project/projected 73, 132; by analyst, onto referrer 45; by child 13, 107; difficult to share 147; experiences 36; externally 3; future 146; hatred 95; internal 133; internal coldness 139; mental death 124; narcissistic mirroring 43; need for help 10; parts 146; by patient, onto analyst 80, 85, 89, 128; return in aggressive form 28; therapeutic, abandoned 113; transference 123
projection(s) 11, 84, 122; connected with exhibitionism 61; continuous use of 30; of Ego 107; fear of death 13; of feelings onto the other 28; infant 64; of one's emotional state 39; patient's 142–143; people masked by 59
projective identification(s) 75, 82, 124; communicative nature of 81; containing activates the process of 41; continuous use of 30; emotional requests made through 150; excessive 10, 44, 63; interpersonal relationship established by utilizing 88; intrusive 18; not used 84; of the past 77; pathological 16; process of 135; role of 27; use of 123
psychic 61; apparatus 31–32; collapse 90; development 26, 101; discomfort 61; economy, disorders in 154; element(s) 18, 32; emptiness and desolation 124; 'I' 120; immobility 95; life 65; meanings 53, 60, 125; parts 45; phenomenon 11, 67; proximity 88; reality, kept at a distance 103; retreat 111, 114; state, immature 66; strength, loss of faith in 75; structure 106; survival 9, 89, 128; transformations 72; trauma 151; world 14, 62
psychic area 7–8; transformations in 99
psychic death 110, 151; imminent 107
psychic experiences 90; of the new-born 106
psychic pain 113; defence against 90
psychic space 14; interior, development of 20; intra- 14
psychic survival 9, 89, 128
psychoanalytical: intervention 8; work 7
psychoanalytic myth 101; observation 118; practice 121; process 9; psychotherapy 2, 100; study of patients with eczema 61; theories 148, 150; trajectory 4
psychoanalytic work 7; with *desaffectés* 3; hampered by psychic retreat 114
psychosis/psychoses 2, 7, 57, 94, 149
psychosomatic 15; flood of fear 30; forms 70; illnesses 123; medicine 51; patients 129; personalities 8; processes 31; symptoms 1–2, 10, 12, 99
psychosomatic disorders 29–30, 62, 84, 90, 94, 134, 136
psychotic 1; anxieties reappear 81; children 57, 80; crisis 102; episode of depersonalization 94; mental state 74; mother 99, 104; neurotic-psychotic mode 53; nuclei 11; person 14; psychological organization 8; symptomatology, initial 99; symptoms 94
psychotic parts 130, 144; hatred of 128
psychotic patients 34, 65, 94, 114, 119; patients 26; adult 13, 57
psychotics 13–14
psychotic structures 154; psychological 8
pudore 126–127

reclaim 85; need to be reclaimed 125; reclamation 64, 138
Reed, G.S. 11–12, 21n2, 130
Reiner, A. 21n2, 92
rejection 117; acceptance without 96;

Index

aesthetic impact 45; affectionate feelings replaced by 92; attempts to escape 112; danger of 43; desire to receive love and attention 15; distance denotes 16; of end to relationship with analyst 147; experience transformed 136; feelings of 104, 110; gesture of 106; masked 10; outwardly displayed 95; patient hypersensitive to 77; patterns may emerge 34; reactions triggered by analyst's rules 104; self 108; tone expressive of 119; towards intelligence 100

relationship(s) 15, 18, 30, 32, 39, 54, 56, 78, 87, 89, 119, 138; absence of feelings in 100; of affection 46; based on control 58; beauty 42–44; confusion in 53; continue 112–113; continuity in 149, 151; defensive withdrawal from 125; denial of 97; desire for 141; develop feelings in 34; development of 155; development prevented 120; ended 74, 84; escaping responsibility in 65; establish by imitation 83; with external mother 107; family 111; fusional 9, 17; with grandmother 150; helpful 69; hindered 29; human 3, 13, 41, 56–57, 75, 77, 151; importance of surface 70; internalized 105; lack of meaning in 36; loss of beautiful aspects 71; meaning 90, 146; new-born artificial 52; obsessive collection of 79; parasite-host or *folie-à-deux* 28; primitive 92, 95, 108; primitive fears regarding 12; problems with real 98; problems, source of 109; productive 46, 118; professional 112; re-enactment in 9, 124; rejection of 12, 15; sexual 59, 62, 72; between space and time 20; stable 75, 106; tattoos 28; therapeutic 4, 45, 54, 57, 99, 111; threats in 85, 133; transference 4, 95; transference through 123; transference/countertransference 151; unconscious 107–108; unstable 106

relationship(s), affective 2, 100; addictions in lieu of 127; adult 108; analytic work around 106; attempting to initiate 143; autistic structure prevented 95; difficulty in 104; established 145; interpersonal 84; with patient 82, 86; personal dilemma 102; reduced 10; separating 147; strengthened 135; success in 136

relationship(s), analytic 3, 9, 76, 80, 110, 134, 137, 144; adhesive identification in 36; adhesiveness 59, 77, 122; atmosphere of profound affection in 82; communication in 7; difficulties in 133; duration 146; effort to stay in 104; enabled to unfold 113; intimacy of 57; past behaviours as weapon to destroy 85; with patient 152; static nature of 111; storyline for development 120; strengthened 144; on two tracks 82

relationship(s), emotional 43; contain and process 129; difficulty in establishing 55; interpersonal 121; stable 9; unattainable 127

relationship(s), interpersonal 3, 64–65, 137; anxiety when establishing 15; autism involves immobility in 143; characterized by mania and omnipotence 128; consolidated 146; controlled 103; difficulties with 60; dominant role of sight in 53; emotional 121; inability to attribute feelings of love to 136; with mother 103; negation of 97; profound 62, 73; projective identification 88; superficial 55; transforming 143; try to avoid 134

relationship(s), object 62; absence of 9; allergic 30; characterized by violence 44; children unable to establish 96; dimensions of 40; establishment of 11; existed only in presence of the other 74; internal 107; lack of 124; normality implies existence of 84; patient's primitive experience of 122; pudore connected to 127; two-dimensional 41; type of 18

relationship(s) parent-infant 13; mother-child 16–17, 89, 97, 111, 119; pathological 67

relationship between skin and Self 26; and early sensory experiences 1; and problems of identity 28; of Self and skin of the other 20

repeat/repeated/repeating 9, 72, 84; acting-out 80; autistic activities 73; behaviours showing aggression 64; caresses 73; fantasies/phantasies 91, 95; frustrations 12; intrusion of a bad object 130; movements (of robots) 98; nasal sounds 61; patients ask the therapist to 144; patterns 85; same subject (chuntering) 144; sensory experiences 33; through transference 124

repetition 111; of autistic activities 62; of defence mechanisms 122; obsessive 61; of partial and irregular dis-investment 12; of the past 120; relinquishing 136; of sensations 66
repetitive behaviour 139, 145; autistic manoeuvres 134, 136; caresses 62; elements shared with others 70; meaningless 123, 135; organization 123
Resnik, S. 52, 60, 84, 118–119, 148, 150
reverie 7, 56–57
robots 98; robot-like 33–34
Rosenfeld, D. 26–29, 61, 150
Rosenfeld, H. 7

sadistic: attacks 10, 80, 111; feelings evoked 127, 151; messages 85; transference 59
Sami-Ali, M. 30
Scarfone, D. 21n2
Schur, M. 30, 61
scratching 30, 61; itchingscratching cycle 30
second skin 27; with adhesive qualities 41; different solutions to a failure 32; formation of 29, 33
Segal, H. 18, 20
Self 8, 36, 51; acceptance of separation 127; acknowledges need for authentic 147; acquired over time 51; analyst looks within 124; addiction as escape from thinking of 135, 145; aggression towards 28; apparently structured 55, 60; appearance as representation of 26; autistic-type capsules buried in 8; concept of space 41; death of, in early stages of life 90; death of meanings of 13; desire to kill 65; emotional needs 18; evolution towards new way of life 147; false 52, 120; felt to be worthless 12; harmonious, lacked 100; 'I' created later 51; integration of 2, 154; isolation of potential 34; language connected to deepest meaning of 51; mother's 43–44; non-being 55, 62; premature establishment 133; primitive identification with It 51; recognition of 19; relationship with skin of the other 20; surfaces of 35; terror of losing integrity of 94; time absent as internal coordinate of 145; took possession of 100; true 52, 120, 154; *see also* new Self, own Self

Self in children: damaged 138; psychological 16; patient's child-like aspects 81
Self confusion 9; in sense of 87; regarding limits of 54
Self, construction of 1, 12; defensive, to simulate 120
Self, deficits in 3, 53; defective formation of 14; deficiency of 65, 80; traumatic experiences responsible for 53
Self, development of 26, 99, 154; degree of, psychoanalytical intervention appropriate for 8
enriched by time 41; development of sense of 17, 29; theory 106
Self dissolution/disintegration: crisis of 149, 154; symptoms of 74
Self, experience of: primitive, recall impedes change 14; traumatic, responsible for deficits in 53; surface with no inner space 35, 40
Self, non-existent 64; partial 60
Self objects 90; bad, presence of 12; no interest in internal 44
Self protection: from non-Self 119; inside the other 18
Self, sense of: confusion in 87; development of 17, 29; stronger 29
self-analysis 54; completed only with the patient's help 133; constant 113; continuous 155; need for 132; stimulating greater depth in 44
self-image 39, 52, 137
Self, part(s) of the 3, 7, 12, 14; experience of losing 107; fragility of 103; hidden 1; missing 55; more evolved side of 18; object to contain 33; object to support 35; problematic 133; reveal 52; skin containing 31, 34; unconscious relationships between 107; wants to return to passive position of victim 65
self-rejection 108
Selz, M. 126
sensory experiences: addiction to 55; early 1, 55, 62; immediate (through sight) 38, 46; lack of symbolization of 18; mental representation of skin linked to 31; primitive 43, 84; repeated 33; unprocessed 8, 84
separation 59–60, 85, 129; acceptance as space between Self and other 127; accepting feelings regarding 141; acknowledgement prevented 123;

Index

adhesive identification does not permit 124; anxiety 15; from autistic state 86; brings up fantasies 147; concepts of space and time emerge at 20; defended self by devaluating other person 71; feeling pain about upcoming 113; final 147; happening too abruptly or completely 32; help patient bear 122; inability to acknowledge bodily 66; like tearing away part of body surface from other's 71; mourning of 82; not processed 9, 103; orifices represent 62; from outside world, lack of 33; patients with dermatological ailments facing 30; patients unable to endure 20; premature 19; processing prevented by obsessive ideation 127; progress in analysis is beginning of 146; suffering subsequent to 28; in symbiosis, equivalent to disintegration 17; time of 141

separation experience 30, 59, 124; as final disappearance of other 135, 143; occurs at skin level 30; past, anger over re-living 75; previous 139; represents loss 147; subjectivity emerges from 143; as threat of abandonment 15

separation process 19; acknowledged 146; felt as attack 32; promote 89

shell 70; in dreams 70, 87; Ego- 18; illusory skin 28; type personality 33

sight 40; blurred 76; control by 18; as controlling mechanism 82; disconnected from thinking 33; dominant role 53; enjoyment that comes from 42; fear of losing control through 103; knowledge about the other gained through 118; love at first sight 39; noble sense 38; pleasure given by 70; primacy 38; sensory experiences 43, 46; summarizes person as a whole 119; surrogate for touch 15; *see also* at first sight

skin 21, 27, 41, 60, 69; absence of containment by 67; aggression towards others 61; in autism 29; beautiful 68; boundaries represented by 18; colour of 117; common 32; conceptualization of 26; as container 154; containment by 73; containment offered 62; covering the face 119; deterioration of 94; discomfort shifted onto 61; dreams about 71–72, 87; Ego-skin 32; erotogenic zone 33, 61; experience of separation 30; first place of exchange 31; frightened at the changes in 94; importance in experiences of autistic states 3; loss of 87; malformations of 71; need to change 88; over-stimulation of 32; primitive experience of 18; shedding 88; shield 33; provides containment 71; psychic transformations 72; response to sensations felt 36; role of 35, 70, 87; role in development of psychic apparatus 31–32; of Self/other 20; sensations 33; skinless hole 63; surface, experience of 34–35; tattoos 28; unconscious mental representation of 31; *see also* second skin

skin contact 62, 72; first experiences 35; physical 89; superficial 15

skin diseases and disorders 15, 26, 34; allergic 29–30; eczema 123; inflammation of 30; irritation 31; problems 61; suffering transferred to 1, 28

skin functions 34; containing 35; first 87; of individuation 33; protective sensory meaning 72

skin as organ 55; of expression 31; of action, primitive 53

skin in relationship with: abandoning relationships 15; clothes 26; development of Self 26; early sensory experiences 1; emotional changes visible through 27; identity 27; others 15; problems of identity 28; psychic development 26; Self and of Other 20

somatic *see* psychosomatic

Spitz, R. 11, 30

Steiner, J. 114, 136

suicidal thoughts 63, 151

suicide: phantasies of 105; threat of 85

surface(s) 1, 28, 56, 59, 62, 84; contact with other 40; cutaneous 40; dreams about 69–70; evaluation 18; external aspects of 26; fascination of 70; impossible to internalize 79; interest in 40; living on the 28, 33; maternal 36; meaning of 35, 40; of the other 36; outer 34; outer active 31; patients' interest in 26; of people and objects 70; pleasure given by 70; Self as 34; sensitive qualities of 40; sensory qualities of 35; tearing away part of 71; theme of 26; without depth 71

surface(s), skin: aggression located on 61; of the body 31, 33–35, 79, 94; child's bodily 41

symbiotic: fantasies 141; fusion 62; identity 30; relationships 59; stage 15
Symington, N. 65, 81, 100–101, 110, 128

terror 45; of bodily sensations 29; crises of 95; of disconnection with mother 66; dreams full of 68; of dying 29; of emptiness 90; episodes of 8; existential 149, 154; of falling into limitless and formless space 9; feelings of 29; of having separate identity 74; of losing integrity of Self 94; of non-being 87; phantasies 105; unnamed/nameless 8, 82
terror experienced: in archaic periods 90; by autistic children 29; represented by black hole 13, 79
therapeutic 11, 154; alliance 154; anti-therapeutic 81; attempts 86; changes 10; contacts 72; couple 135; endeavours resisted 94; factor 151; feelings 150; function relinquished 84; good results impossible 134; help/aid 96, 139; interventions 1–2, 54, 109, 130, 142, 149; journeys 4, 94, 100, 147; medical surgery 46; project abandoned 113; reflections on oneself 155; relationship 4, 45, 54, 57, 95, 99, 111, 118; research tool 10; situation, development of 80; tool 148; undertaking 82; work 2–3, 65, 148–149
therapist(s) 3–4, 58, 152; act of reclamation by 138; differences in personality of 118; fear evoked fear in 128; feelings of love and hate towards 121; fill in alpha function 125; female 56; need to be firm in the role 127; plasticity allows continuous adaptations 155; practices patience and perseverance 114; question self-confidence as 80; reconsider previous hypotheses 113; relationship with 123; repetition 144; role as 56; tries to take on and develop meaningful significances 144; use of imagination 125
time and space 54, 129; contact seeming to exist beyond 62; difficulty in respecting 14; transformation of concept of 143
transference 104, 110; adaptations to variations in 155; aggression in 77, 135; brings to light confusing messages 121; communication taking place 149; continuous monitoring of 155; countertransference relationship 151; difficulties in 9; difficult to speak about 74; double 150; experience 97; fluctuations/vicissitudes of 2, 4, 59–60, 122; happens through the object 11; hatred and rejection placed in 119; initial 56, 95; irritation/contempt expressed 73; making the other powerless to help 129; mental construction based on primitive experiences 121; modifications shown in dreams 78; negative 123, 125, 129; recreates deadly trauma 125; relationship, explanation sought 95; repeats primitive emotions 124; starts at initial observation 118
transference, changes in 9; from fight to union 73; from start to finish 100
transference/countertransference relationship 151
transference, interpretations of 91, 146; impossible 96
transference by patient 7, 54; onto analyst 85; into analyst's body 123; feelings experienced by analyst in response to 149; therapist as representative of patient's parents 121; used to provoke reaction 122–123
trauma 113, 151; initial 114, 151; transference recreates 125
Tremelloni, L. 1, 7–8, 12, 34, 45, 94
Tustin, F. 1, 7–8, 10, 13–15, 18, 20, 29, 33–34, 62, 66, 73, 83, 88, 92n1, 127, 134–135
two-dimensional 35; autistic world 35, 40, 88; defensive operation 41; interaction with objects 36, 41; primitive experience 124

Ulnik, J. 15, 26, 30, 53, 61
un-mentalized: experiences 8, 55; parts 86

weakness 13, 35; acceptance of 99; bodily experiences of 90; image of 123; mistaking love for 78; patience as a sign of 134; of patient's representations of primary object 149; perception of one's own 146
Winnicott, D.W. 7–8, 10–13, 18–19, 30, 52, 59, 129, 133